Women, oppression and social work

Issues in anti-discriminatory practice

Much of the progress achieved by the women's movement now seems threatened by the combined effects of prolonged economic insecurity, reductions in the scope of welfare provision and a general shift in the climate of public opinion to the right. Consequently, social workers are faced with the growing demands of a more impoverished and unstable society, with diminishing resources to meet these demands.

In response to these pressures, feminist social work has begun to move beyond some of the limitations of both the traditional and radical social work models of the past. The emerging anti-discriminatory model recognises the diversity of oppressions according to race, gender and class as well as those of age, disability and sexual orientation.

Women, Oppression and Social Work offers a new perspective on feminist social work which takes account of the complexity of the manifold oppressions that affect the lives of most women and most social work clients. It will be valuable reading for all professionals in training and in practice, and undergraduates and lecturers in social work, social policy and women's studies.

Mary Langan lectures in Social Policy at the Open University and **Lesley Day** lectures in Sociology and Social Policy at the West London Institute of Higher Education.

The State of Welfare
Edited by Mary Langan

Nearly half a century after its post-war consolidation, the British Welfare state is once again at the centre of political controversy. After a decade in which the role of the state in the provision of welfare was steadily reduced in favour of the private, voluntary and informal sectors, with relatively little public debate or resistance, the further extension of the new mixed economy of welfare in the spheres of health and education became a major political issue in the early 1990s. At the same time the impact of deepening recession has begun to expose some of the deficiencies of market forces in areas, such as housing and income maintenance, where the role had expanded dramatically during the 1980s. *The State of Welfare* provides a forum for continuing the debate about the services we need in the 1990s.

Titles of Related Interest

Also in *The State of Welfare Series*

The Dynamics of British Health Policy
Stephen Harrison, David Hunter, Christopher Pollitt

Ideologies of Welfare: from Dreams to Disillusion
John Clarke, Ian Cochrane, Carol Smart

Managing Poverty
Carol Walker

Radical Social Work Today
Edited by Mary Langan, Phil Lee

Taking Child Abuse Seriously
The Violence Against Children Study Group

Women, oppression and social work

Issues in anti-discriminatory practice

Edited by

Mary Langan and Lesley Day

Routledge
Taylor & Francis Group
LONDON AND NEW YORK

First published 1992 by Routledge

2 Park Square, Milton Park, Abingdon, Oxon OX14 4RN
711 Third Avenue, New York, NY 10017, USA

Routledge is an imprint of the Taylor & Francis Group, an informa business

First issued in hardback 2016

Transferred to Digital Printing 2005

Typeset by Fotographics (Bedford) Ltd

A Tavistock/Routledge Publication

British Library Cataloguing in Publication Data
A catalogue record for this book is available from the British Library

Library of Congress Cataloguing in Publication Data
A catalogue record for this book is available from the Library of Congress

ISBN 0-415-08030-4 (hbk) ISBN 0-415-07611-0 (pbk)

ISBN 978-0-415-07611-1 (pbk)
ISBN 978-1-138-15596-1 (hbk)

Contents

Acknowledgement

Although this book began with joint and equal editorship, Mary Langan has undertaken the bulk of the editorial work, keeping the project alive and providing support and guidance to most of the contributors. I would like to acknowledge this and express my thanks for her perseverance and patience.

Lesley Day

Contributors

Cathy Aymer is principal lecturer in social work at the West London Institute of Higher Education, and is the course leader of a large social work course. She has spent several years in residential work with young people, both as a basic grade worker and as a unit manager. She is currently involved in training and consultancy in the areas of staff team building, work with girls and young men, anti-racist practice and management training. She is a black woman and is particularly interested in issues of race, gender and sexuality in social work education and practice.

Helen Cosis Brown works as a lecturer in social work at Middlesex Polytechnic. She worked for nine years in the London Borough of Camden social services department as a social worker and a team leader. As well as lecturing she works as a freelance trainer and consultant in the area of gender, and on issues of sexual orientation relevant to social work practice. She is currently undertaking research, jointly with Jenny Pearce (Middlesex Polytechnic), on young women and the implications for social work practice of the Children Act, 1989.

Agnes Bryan was born in Grenada; she has a MA in organizational analysis from Birkbeck College and is presently a senior lecturer in social work at the West London Institute of Higher Education. She has worked for several years in the community social work and adult education/training fields. She is committed to working with black women and has long experience of work with black community groups. She is at present engaged in research on the experience of women and black people in senior positions in educational institutions.

Pam Carter is a white woman who lectures in social policy in the Department of Economics and Government and with the Social Welfare Research Unit at Newcastle upon Tyne Polytechnic. She has extensive experience of teaching social work both in higher education and as a practice teacher. With Tony Jeffs and Mark Smith she edits the *Social Work and Social Welfare Yearbook*. She is currently researching into women's experiences of infant feeding.

Lesley Day is senior lecturer in sociology and social policy in the Department of Social Work at the West London Institute of Higher Education. She was previously research and policy adviser at the Personal Social Services Council. She has been involved in the field of Intermediate Treatment for some years and published in the area of policies for young women and men in trouble. She is also a member of the editorial collective of *Critical Social Policy*. Currently, she is training to be a counsellor and hopes in the future to combine teaching with establishing a counselling service for women in the West London area.

Angela Everitt is a white woman, currently reader in social welfare studies and responsible for the Social Welfare Research Unit at Newcastle upon Tyne Polytechnic. She has been involved in social work education in both teaching and management. She has published on women in management and is currently completing a book on practitioner research with Pauline Hardiker, Jane Littlewood and Audrey Mullinder.

Annie Hudson is a team manager working in central Bristol for Avon social services department. A white woman, she was formerly employed as a lecturer in social work at the University of Manchester, where she had particular research and teaching interests in work with young women, child abuse, social work management and in developing feminist perspectives on social work.

Beverley Hughes is a white British woman, who qualified as a probation officer (CQSW) in 1974. After several years in practice, she completed two major DHSS-funded research projects, one concerned with the residential care of old people. Now a lecturer in social work at Manchester University, she has published various articles concerned with older people, including work on residential care, health and quality of life. With Melody Mtezuka she has developed specialist training courses for social workers and students on social work with older people, based on a critical gerontological perspective.

Mary Langan is a lecturer in social policy at the Open University. She has extensive experience of social work and social work education and is currently involved in developing open and distance learning techniques in social policy and social work education. Her research interests include the relationship between the state, social policy and social work, equal opportunities and social work, and comparative social policy in Europe. Her publications include *Crises* *in the British State 1880–1930* (with Bill Schwarz, Hutchinson, 1985), *Radical Social Work Today* (with Phil Lee, Unwin Hyman, 1989). She is General Editor of the Harper Collins social policy series *The State of Welfare*.

Marilyn Lawrence trained and worked as a psychiatric social worker. She has held lectureships in social work at the University of Bradford and the West London Institute of Higher Education. Since 1980 she has been involved in the educational work of The Women's Therapy Centre. She is a white woman who now works as a psychotherapist and is senior clinical lecturer in social work at the Tavistock Clinic. Her published works include *The Anorexic Experience* (1984), *Fed Up and Hungry* (1987) and with Mira Dana, *Women's Secret Disorder* (1988) and *Fighting Food* (1990).

Carol Lupton is currently senior research officer and acting head of the Social Services Research and Information Unit, Portsmouth Polytechnic. Her main research and publications have been in the areas of feminist research practice, policy development within the personal social services and quality assurance in community care services. She is currently editing a book on the dilemmas and compromises of feminist practice. She serves on the editorial board of *Research Policy and Planning*, the Journal of the Social Services Research Group, and regularly abstracts on feminist research and social work practice for *Women's Abstracts*.

Marie McNay is principal lecturer in social work at the School of Social and Historical Studies, Portsmouth Polytechnic. Prior to that, she worked as a senior lecturer in social work at the Polytechnic of Central London and the West London Institute of Higher Education. She has worked in several local authority social service departments and in a psychiatric hospital. Her professional interests include family work and community oriented social work and trade unionism. Her previous publications are The *Concept of Groupwork in the Field of Social Work* (Psychiatric Rehabilitation Association, 1969) and *Low Pay and Family Poverty* (with co-author, Chris Pond, Study Commission on the Family, 1980).

Melody Mtezuka is a black South African woman and she obtained her social work qualifications in Zambia and England. She has practised mainly in child guidance where she developed an interest in examining how people from black and ethnic minority backgrounds were treated within social work agencies in Britain. Since joining the Department of Social Policy at Manchester University as a lecturer she has developed her critique of the lack of anti-racist strategies in social work practice. She has also researched and is about to publish on the subject of child sexual abuse among ethnic minority families and she is developing her interest in older people from black and ethnic minorities.

Fiona Williams lives in Leeds and is a lecturer in the Department of Health and Social Welfare at the Open University. Her publications include *Social Policy: A Critical Introduction, Issues of Race, Gender and Class* (Polity Press, 1989) and she is co-editor of *Know Me As I Am: An Anthology of Prose, Poetry and Art by People with Learning Difficulties* (Hodder and Stoughton, 1990). She has been involved in the socialist and feminist and anti-racist movements for many years and is on the editorial collective of *Critical Social Policy*.

Series editor's preface

Within days of Margaret Thatcher's dramatic resignation as Conservative Party leader and prime minister in November 1990, a major study entitled *The State of Welfare*, carried out at the London School of Economics on behalf of the Economic and Social Research Council, concluded that the Thatcher years 'had failed to roll back the welfare state' (Hills 1990). The authors showed that though total spending on welfare as a proportion of all public expenditure declined in the mid-1980s from the 55.7 per cent level it reached in 1977–8 under Labour, it had risen again to 55.6 per cent by 1987–8. Welfare spending as a proportion of GDP followed a parallel course: 22.9 per cent in 1979–80, 23.2 per cent in 1987–8. These figures appeared to support the view that, despite the anti-welfare rhetoric of the right and the protests over 'the cuts' from the left, the welfare state had emerged largely unscathed from the Thatcher decade.

Yet global figures on welfare spending conceal as much as they reveal. The view that a consistent level of spending guarantees a consistent level of service rests on the assumption that the level of need also remains constant. However, all the evidence suggests that the 1980s was a decade in which there was a rising level of need for welfare services in British society. This increase in demand came not from insatiable welfare professionals, profligate bureaucrats or greedy consumers, but from the real needs of a steadily rising population of older people, a now permanent reserve army of labour, at least two million strong, and a growing body of the low paid and poor. Constant welfare spending during a period of rising demand means deteriorating services and deteriorating benefits for a substantial and growing section of the population.

Global figures also conceal significant variations among different sections of welfare. During the 1980s there was a dramatic increase in spending on social security or income maintenance, largely as a result of the persistent unemployment throughout the decade. Here the overall increase in spending concealed a general stagnation in the purchasing power of benefits and a significant decline in the value of certain benefits, notably old age pensions and child benefit. The figures also fail to reveal the effect of measures to exclude many young people from any right to claim benefits and the consequent appearance of young beggars on a large scale in British cities.

Expenditure on health also showed an overall increase, but this was scarcely enough to meet the health-care needs of more older people, to make new techniques such as organ transplantation widely available, or to allow the health service to cope with the consequences of new problems such as HIV infection and Aids.

Other spheres of welfare – notably in education and housing – registered significant cuts in public spending. The results in education have been a chronic demoralization of staff and a series of disputes at every level from nurseries to universities. The mass privatization of council housing and the virtual cessation of public housing construction have resulted in the emergence of homelessness as a major national scandal. By the end of 1990 it was estimated that four to five thousand people were sleeping on the streets, two to three thousand in London alone.

Statistics that show a steady level of welfare spending also fail to reveal the differential impact of the restructuring of welfare services through the 1980s. The LSE/ESRC study noted how middle-class people were relatively favoured by the shifts in the pattern of expenditure:

> All the services which grew at the same rate as, or faster than, need are those which benefit the middle classes at least as much as, if not more than, the less well-off; all those which fell relative to need, except for higher education, are those in which the middle classes have little or no stake (LeGrand 1990: 346).

Thus, behind the apparent resilience of the welfare state lies the reality of a system of benefits and services which has been rationalized and restructured in such a way that it fails to meet the real needs of British society and fails most those in the greatest need.

In his early days as prime minister, John Major suggested that he might offer a less abrasive approach towards the welfare state than his predecessor. Not only did he proclaim his commitment to creating 'a classless society', but his new ministerial team stepped up the provision of hostels for the young homeless in London, made an out of court settlement with haemophiliacs infected with HIV, backed away from a direct link between the assessment of teachers' performance and their pay levels and even admitted to having overdone the 'language of commerce' in its approach to health service reforms.

Yet the British government moves into the 1990s with the unmistakable signs of deepening recession ahead. The inevitable response of any government committed to maintaining the profitability of private enterprise will be to curtail still further expenditure on welfare. The effects of privatization and market reforms in the health service, education and all spheres of central and local government have already moved beyond mere rhetoric to dictate the restructuring of services according to the needs of the market. It is difficult to avoid the conclusion that for the poor, for women, for older people, for black people and members of ethnic minorities, for people with disabilities or learning difficulties, and for all those who work in the field of welfare, there will be even harder times in the 1990s.

Mary Langan
January 1991

References

Hills, J. (ed.) (1990), *The State of Welfare: The Welfare State in Britain Since 1990* (Oxford: Oxford University Press).
LeGrand, J. (1990), 'The state of welfare', in Hills 1990, pp. 338–62.

Introduction: women and social work in the 1990s

Mary Langan

These are difficult times for women and difficult times too for social work. Many of the gains of the women's movement over the past twenty years now seem threatened by the combined effects of prolonged economic insecurity, reductions across the board in the scope of public welfare provision, and a general shift in the climate of opinion in a more conservative direction. Persistent unemployment and declining living standards for low-income households since the mid-1970s have led to steadily rising poverty for a substantial section of the British population. Over the same period income-maintenance benefit levels have declined in real terms, public housing has been drastically reduced by council-house sales, and health and education services have slowly deteriorated.

An increasing burden of all aspects of welfare has been pushed back onto women in the home. Local government – the main provider of social work services – has been a particular target of central government political attack and financial constraint. The restructuring of public services according to the dictates of market forces, accompanied by a fierce ideological offensive against the more liberal policies of the post-war decades, have transformed the world of welfare. Social workers are faced with the growing demands of a more elderly, more impoverished and more unstable society. They have fewer resources with which to meet these demands, and they are forced to work in the face of apparently unrelenting public hostility.

Yet not only has social work survived, but feminist social work has begun to move beyond some of the limitations of both the traditional and the radical social work models of the past. In recent years, feminists have attempted to develop a wider, non-oppressive, anti-discriminatory form of social work theory and practice. This approach questions both the conservative presumptions of orthodox casework, and the simple class and gender frameworks advanced by the radical social work movement, and indeed by the early women's movement. The new approach recognizes the complexity and diversity of the manifold oppressions that affect the lives of most women and most social work clients.

Beginning from the debates between gender and class perspectives in the 1970s, the movement towards anti-discriminatory social work really took off from the encounter between feminist and anti-racist women in the 1980s. It broadened out through the inclusion of the critiques of women of different ethnic, national, religious and cultural identities as well as those of lesbians, women with disabilities and older women. The result has been the emergence of a literature which attempts to establish some principles for anti-discriminatory practice. This book is both a result of, and a contribution to, these experiences and debates. It seeks to identify the essential elements of a feminist, non-oppressive, anti-discriminatory practice for the 1990s.

Origins

Social work emerged in Britain in the post-war decades out of diverse forms of private philanthropic and public welfare interventions in the lives of needy and delinquent children, families in crisis, and other categories of people in need (Younghusband 1978; Younghusband 1981). Given the high level of public confidence that the conditions created by national economic expansion and the establishment of the welfare state had removed poverty and deprivation, those who were unable to cope in society were regarded as suffering from some form of personal inadequacy (Langan 1985). The residual difficulties of the beneficent new social order were blamed on a small number of 'problem families' (Clarke, Langan and Lee 1980). Academic authorities in the social sciences appropriated psychoanalytic models to explain the maladaptive behaviour of individuals and family groups (Wilson 1977; Yelloly 1980). Casework techniques were developed to enable expert workers to intervene in order to restore individuals to effective social citizenship (Jones 1983; Jordan 1984).

In the 1970s the individualistic approach and casework methods of traditional social work came under challenge from the radical social work movement (Bailey and Brake 1975; Brake and Bailey 1980). In circumstances of rising unemployment and growing austerity, radical social workers emphasized the structural determinants of deviant behaviour in society. Often strongly influenced by Marxist or socialist ideas, they drew attention to the overwhelmingly working-class character of social work clients. They insisted that an analysis of the oppressive social relationships endured by these clients was essential to understand their responses to society.

Furthermore they emphasized that the practice of social work as a means to correct clients' adjustment to an oppressive social reality was both futile and politically unjustifiable. They advocated a collective approach to the resolution of social problems, through working with tenants' groups, community associations, trade unions and other organizations of working-class people (Corrigan and Leonard 1978; Bolger *et al.* 1981; Jones 1983).

In the course of the 1980s the limitations of both the traditional and the radical models became increasingly apparent, especially to feminist social workers. The women's movement had emerged alongside the development of radical social work, and became increasingly critical of its narrow analytic framework and the restricted scope of its approach to practice (Langan and Lee 1989). As a product of the established left, the radical social work movement was male-dominated and often insensitive to some of the basic realities of the world of social work, notably the fact that the large majority of both clients and workers are women (Brook and Davis 1985).

Feminist social workers drew attention to the role of patriarchal power relations in all spheres, from the families of clients to the hierarchy of social services departments, and emphasized the need to raise awareness of these relations and to challenge them (Marchant and Wearing 1986; Hanmer and Statham 1988; Dominelli and McLeod 1989; Hallett 1989). Both from within the women's movement, and from autonomous organizations of black people and those of other ethnic minorities, came further demands that the world of social work acknowledge the diversity of oppression in British society and organize to tackle it (Rooney 1982; Ahmed, Cheetham and Small 1986; Hughes and Bhaduri 1987; Rooney 1987; Dominelli 1988; Roys 1988). Social work has also been obliged to become aware of discrimination on grounds of age (Phillipson 1989) and disability (Lonsdale 1990).

The attempt to construct an anti-discriminatory social work has taken shape out of a growing recognition of the specificities of oppression, according to gender, race, class, age, disability and sexual orientation (Langan and Lee 1989). It emphasizes the diversity of experience and the validity of each person's experience. It seeks to develop an understanding of both the totality of oppression and its specific manifestations as the precondition for developing an anti-discriminatory practice relevant to all spheres of social work.

'Difference'

Whereas the early women's movement emphasized the inequalities between women and men, new theories of difference question these gender categories and emphasize diversity *within* the concept of 'woman', which, for feminist analysis, had previously been accepted as a unitary category. The feminist claim to represent the interests of all women was first challenged by the traditional left, which pointed to profound class differences and antagonisms among women. Any universal claims of the women's movement were undermined by the critique by black feminists of the implicit ethnocentrism and racism of the movement's assumptions. Further contributions from lesbians, older women and women with disabilities helped to bury the old simplicities and contributed to the emergence of more diverse forms of 'pluralistic' feminism. These developments corresponded with the wider rejection, by those influenced by post-structuralist and post-modernist theories, of the notion of a unified subject as the agent of social or political change.

As Michelle Barrett has argued, distinct and to some extent contradictory, theories of difference have emerged. On the one hand, there is the emphasis on 'experiential diversity', an approach which corresponds to a long-standing feminist tradition. On the other hand, there is the post-modernist conception of difference as 'positional meaning'. From a perspective that rejects the possibility of any 'transcendental' meaning or purpose, in favour of emphasizing meanings constructed through necessarily fragmented discourses, there can be no *common* political project for women (Barrett 1987).

Both these theories of difference may be criticized for encouraging intellectual and political separatism and fragmentation. The emphasis on individual experience may be further criticized as taking experience itself for granted, for underestimating the way in which all experience is mediated through received ideas and inherently ideological frameworks of thought. This in turn leads to the criticism that 'experiential diversity' implies a relativist view of knowledge and a moralistic political discourse: the specificity of each woman's experience is assumed to guarantee its authenticity and legitimacy. The price for encouraging such a concept of diversity may well be the loss of coherence in the women's movement and the abandonment of any project of collective resistance. This abandonment of any commitment to change and any agency through which it can be achieved also appears to be the outcome of theories of 'positional meaning'.

Thus, though we can recognize the importance of the divisions among women, some current conceptions of difference give rise to difficulties. How, for example, can we move beyond recognizing 'difference' to understanding the interconnections among different groups of women, to grasping what we have in common? As Mary Maynard writes: 'Just as it has been argued that gender cannot be simply added on to class analysis, so too it is mistaken to just add race on to existing analyses of gender' (Maynard 1990: 281). Race does not simply make the experience of women's subordination greater, it qualitatively changes the nature of that subordination. However, while different oppressions interact and reinforce one another, emphasizing 'difference' *per se* may lead to division and conflict.

Another debate is taking place among feminists, between those who favour jettisoning 'woman' as an analytic category and those who regard it as crucial for the study of gender differences (Delmar 1986; Mitchell 1986; Maynard 1990). Many would probably agree with Maynard that recognizing the diversity among women should not detract from recognizing the concept of 'woman' and the major significance of the imbalance in power relations between women and men in the organization of society. She endorses Ramazanoglu's view that feminists should work with the contradiction that women are simultaneously united as a group and also divided (Ramazanoglu 1989). Feminists should focus more on what is required to liberate them rather than on what oppresses them. This involves challenging the nature of power, whoever holds it, including being sensitive to the power some women have over other women, and the need, for example, for white feminists to confront their own racism. This approach places a greater emphasis on the active, resisting role of women as opposed to their passive role as victims of power relations, offers a constructive resolution of the often pessimistic debates of the late 1980s, and points towards a more positive political practice in the 1990s.

The contributors to this book write from a variety of theoretical perspectives within feminism. One of the great strengths of the women's movement has always been the diversity of its debates and its capacity to absorb prevailing intellectual trends into its discourse. The contributors differ on a range of issues; in particular they place varying emphasis on the questions of difference – some identifying more heterogeneity, others less. These divergences reflect the current state of the debate and the quest to define more precisely what unites women as an oppressed group and what divides them. There is a common concern, however, to discover how parallel processes of discrimination can produce shared understandings and a renewed commitment to anti-discriminatory practice.

Analysing oppression

The first three chapters provide broad analytic perspectives on different forms of oppression and offer some guidelines on anti-discriminatory practice. Surveying the debates on race, class and gender, Lesley Day examines the complex ways in which these modalities of oppression interact and affect women's lives. She assesses the contributions of black and white feminists and argues that the class and race positions of women reconstruct their gendered experience. She insists that it is essential to grasp the complexity of these relations in order to understand the position of women social workers, who, as state agents, occupy a contradictory class location, and their clients, for whom questions of family status and employment, as well as simple gender and race definitions, are important.

Marilyn Lawrence discusses the feminist approach to women's psychology, drawing on feminist psychoanalytic literature. She opens up what often appear as highly technical and esoteric debates and draws out the consequences for anti-discriminatory social work practice. She elaborates in particular on the perennial controversy of the mother–daughter relationship. Her chapter tackles a number of important questions. Are psychoanalytic theories universally valid? Are Freudian, or even post-Freudian, categories relevant across class and race divisions? How useful is a specifically feminist psychoanalytic approach in social work practice with women who are black, white or working class? Are there parallels between the psychic experiences of women under patriarchy and black people in a racist society? Marilyn offers case histories to illustrate what women, as social workers or social work clients, have in common in terms of unmet needs. She also raises the difficult problem of mothers who abuse their children.

Marie McNay attempts to construct a theoretical framework to facilitate a more integrated approach to social work practice. Her framework is underpinned by the concept of power relations and her integrated mode of intervention is informed by the concept of the empowerment of the oppressed. Marie uses systems theory to link understandings of different levels of power and to provide a link between theory and practice. Marie's approach draws together a range of theoretical perspectives, using radical, feminist and anti-racist themes in the process of transforming mainstream theory, rather than negating it. She draws on examples from family work and family therapy to show how a mode of intervention based on empowerment can work in practice.

The next three chapters develop the understanding of the differential oppressions of women and of how different processes of discrimination divide and reconstitute the experiences of particular groups. They also explore how groups divided by different experiences of oppression can develop shared understandings and common strategies of resistance in the context of the wider transformation and restructuring of welfare provision.

Mary Langan's chapter on women and social work analyses the transformation of the personal social services. In particular she examines changes in public policy towards the family, as reflected for example in the 1989 Children Act, and assesses the impact of the promotion of the 'mixed economy of welfare' in the wider context of the government's 'community care' policies. What are the consequences for women, in general, and, in particular, for black women, poor women, older women, women with disabilities, and, not least, for women who are social workers?

The issues raised by the restructuring of state responsibility for care and the extension of central control over all aspects of local government are taken further in Carol Lupton's contribution on the 'new managerialism' in social services departments. While acknowledging the potential value of performance measurement or 'quality assurance', Carol questions the values, assumptions and ideologies that inform current managerial strategies. How far do these strategies go in identifying and attempting to overcome the effects of race, class and gender discrimination? Indeed, to what extent do official policies construct and reproduce processes of discrimination? Who decides what is a legitimate performance indicator? What is the quality of the information by which performance is assessed?

Pam Carter, Angela Everitt and Annie Hudson offer a feminist analysis of social work education which elaborates the interconnections between gender and other forms of oppression at a time when social work education is being restructured around the new qualifications of Diploma in Social Work and Certificate in Social Care. They examine the position of women as students, as members of staff and assess the impact of feminism on the social work curriculum. In theory a greater emphasis on practice-based social work education should bring women practice teachers in social work agencies into greater prominence. However, the authors argue that recent changes in social work education are likely to reproduce existing hierarchies and further disadvantage working-class and black women.

There are some signs that the leading bodies in social work education recognize the importance of promoting anti-discriminatory principles. However it remains to be seen whether the radical overhaul of the social work curriculum that is required can proceed in face of the contradictory demands of the new managerialism. The question of whether the principles of anti-discriminatory social work will prevail over the vocationalism currently in vogue remains to be resolved.

Annie Hudson's chapter on child sexual abuse acts as a link between the earlier contributions on the broad themes and concerns of current social work and the rest of the book which is devoted to specific areas of practice. She begins by setting the current wave of public preoccupation with child sexual abuse in a historical context, drawing illuminating parallels with the moral panics about white slavery, child prostitution and incest in the 1880s. The exposure of the scale of child sexual abuse in modern society has largely been achieved by feminists, through the work of rape crisis centres, incest survivors' groups and feminist social workers and doctors. Yet, as Annie notes, the result has been the emergence of a new welfare 'industry' largely dominated by male professionals. Once child sexual abuse became the focus of mass media and general public concern, men moved in to define the terms of the debate and to administer official agencies.

Annie outlines how social work in relation to child sexual abuse can be reclaimed by women working according to feminist principles. In particular she tackles the question of how feminist social workers can develop practices which ensure child protection while not undermining children's rights and those of their parents.

Anti-discriminatory practice

The last five chapters are all concerned with specific oppressions or specific areas of practice. Fiona Williams focuses on one of the most marginalized and oppressed groups, women with learning difficulties. These women are denied basic rights and oppressed through stereotypes which are often reinforced by social workers. Yet they have begun to fight back. Self-help and advocacy groups have promoted empowerment and some social workers have attempted to create a more cooperative relationship between service users and providers. As Fiona points out, people with learning difficulties are not a homogeneous category, but are divided by class, gender, race and age. She examines the effects of converging sexist and racist practices and stereotypes, which are often carried over into social policy, creating a common sense of powerlessness. She also looks at the controversial issues of reproductive rights and sexuality, and caring and dependency.

Agnes Bryan challenges racist myths and stereotypes about Afro-Caribbean mothers in Britain. She argues that social workers need to understand how racism and sexism intersect to shape black women's lives. In particular she emphasizes the importance of grasping the contradictory views about marriage and motherhood that exist in the black community as a result of the experience of oppression. Agnes critically assesses various models of social work intervention among black mothers, and drawing from her own experience with a voluntary project, she illustrates how an anti-racist, gender-sensitive approach can be developed.

Cathy Aymer focuses on the dilemmas facing care workers in the residential sector. Outlining her own experiences as a care worker in a children's home, Cathy discusses the changing roles of care staff in relation to children in care and the contradictory pressures they experience. She explores debates about sexuality and race which have raged in the residential sector in recent years, at a time when the service has become chronically demoralized by cuts and closures.

Helen Cosis Brown examines an issue that has been largely ignored in mainstream, radical and feminist debates on social policy – that of lesbianism. She observes that discrimination against lesbians in social work tends to operate at two levels: either they are ignored, or all their problems are assumed to stem from their sexual orientation. Helen argues that non-discriminatory practice means rejecting stereotypes, and recognizing both the unique experience of every woman and how she perceives her own oppression. Helen surveys social science theory on lesbianism and the record of political struggle around lesbianism, culminating in the campaign against Clause/Section 28 of the 1988 Local Government Act, which banned the 'promotion' of homosexuality by councils. She examines the question of 'coming out' as it affects lesbian social workers, lecturers and students. Helen also looks at two areas of practice in relation to lesbianism – work with older women and child protection. She considers the problems of negotiating multiple oppressions, such as the interaction between racism and homophobia.

In the final chapter, Beverley Hughes and Melody Mtezuka look at social work with older women. They draw attention to the ways in which different forms of oppression both draw older women together and divide them from one another. They emphasize the importance of social workers knowing the personal history of each older woman in their care, so that their interventions can take account of each woman's unique experience. They analyse the effects of recent policy shifts, in particular the trend towards 'community care'. In conclusion they outline a progressive approach to practice based on the principles of anti-discrimination, emphasizing that empowerment is the key concept for translating anti-discriminatory principles into practice.

The emergence of anti-discriminatory social work has inevitably stimulated tensions and conflicts between its supporters and adherents to the established social work models. The resulting controversies have often been heated, particularly at a time of general insecurity within social work as a result of public expenditure cuts and the general squeeze on local government (Bamford 1990). These difficulties have undoubtedly been exacerbated by the intense and often contradictory pressures put on social workers as a result of an apparently continuous series of child abuse scandals, public inquiries and media inquisitions in the late 1980s (The Violence Against Children Study Group 1990). The promotion of a sense of crisis about the family (encouraged by moral panics about one-parent families, child abuse, delinquency and hooliganism) has created a difficult climate in which to develop progressive alternatives to existing models of social work. Yet, as the diverse contributions to this collection illustrate, such alternatives *are* being developed, in the spheres of both theory and practice.

Acknowledgement

Many thanks are due to Ann Boomer for her secretarial, administrative and moral support during this project.

References

Ahmed, S., Cheetham, J., and Small, J. (eds) (1986), *Social Work with Black Children and their Families* (London: Batsford).

Bailey, R., and Brake, M. (eds) (1975), *Radical Social Work* (London: Edward Arnold).

Bamford, T. (1990), *The Future of Social Work* (London: Macmillan Education).

Barrett, M. (1987), 'The concept of difference', *Feminist Review*, 26: pp. 29–42.

Bolger, S., Corrigan, P., Docking, J., and Frost, N. (1981), *Towards Socialist Welfare Work* (London: Macmillan).

Brake, M., and Bailey, R. (eds) (1980), *Radical Social Work and Practice* (London: Edward Arnold).

Brook, E., and Davis, A. (1985), *Women, The Family and Social Work* (London: Tavistock).

Clarke, J., Langan, M., and Lee, P. (1980), 'Social work: the conditions of crisis' in P. Carlen and M. Collison (eds), *Radical Issues in Criminology*, pp. 178–95 (Oxford: Martin Robertson).

Corrigan, P., and Leonard, P. (1978), *Social Work Practice under Capitalism: A Marxist Approach* (London: Macmillan).

Delmar, R. (1986), 'What is Feminism?' in Mitchell, J. and Oakley, A. (eds), *What is Feminism?*, pp. 8–33 (Oxford: Blackwell).

Dominelli, L. (1988), *Anti-Racist Social Work* (London: Macmillan Education).

Dominelli, L., and McLeod, E. (1989), *Feminist Social Work* (London: Macmillan Education).

Hallett, C. (1989), *Women and Social Services Departments* (London: Harvester Wheatsheaf).
Hanmer, J., and Statham, D. (1988), *Women and Social Work: Towards a Woman Centred Practice* (London: Macmillan Education).
Hughes, R. D., and Bhaduri, S. R. (1987), *Social Services for Ethnic Minorities and Race and Culture in Social Service Delivery* (Manchester: DHSS Social Services Inspectorate NW Region).

Jones, C. (1983), *State Social Work and the Working Class* (London: Macmillan).
Jordan, B. (1984), *Social Work* (Oxford: Blackwell).

Langan, M. (1985), 'The unitary approach: a feminist critique', in E. Brook and A. Davis 1985, pp. 3–27.
Langan, M., and Lee, P. (eds) (1989), *Radical Social Work Today* (London: Unwin Hyman).
Lonsdale, S. (1990), *Women and Disability* (London: Macmillan).

Marchant, H., and Wearing, B. (eds) (1986), *Gender Reclaimed: Women in Social Work* (Sydney: Hale and Iremonger).
Maynard, M. (1990), 'The Reshaping of Sociology? Trends in the Study of Gender', *Sociology*, 24, 2: 269–90.
Mitchell, J. (1986), 'Reflections on Twenty Years of Feminism', in J. Mitchell and A. Oakley 1985, pp. 34–48.

Phillipson, C. (1989), 'Challenging dependency: towards a new social work with older people', in M. Langan and P. Lee 1989, pp. 192–207.

Ramazanoglu, C. (1989), *Feminism and the Contradictions of Oppression* (London: Routledge).
Rooney, B. (1982), 'Black social workers in white departments', in J. Cheetham (ed.), *Social Work and Ethnicity* pp. 184–96 (London: NISW/George Allen and Unwin).
Rooney, B. (1987), *Racism and resistance to change: A study of the black social workers' project, Liverpool Social Services Department 1975–1985* (Liverpool: Department of Sociology, University of Liverpool).
Roys, P. (1988), 'Social Services', in A. Bhat, R. Carr-Hill and S. Ohri (eds), *Britain's Black Population: A New Perspective* 2nd Edition pp. 208–36 (Aldershot: Gower).

Violence Against Children Study Group (eds) (1990), *Taking Child Abuse Seriously* (London: Unwin Hyman).

Wilson, E. (1977), *Women and the Welfare State* (London: Tavistock).

Yelloly, M. A. (1980), *Social Work Theory and Psychoanalysis* (Wokingham: Van Nostrand Reinhold).
Younghusband, E. (1978), *Social Work in Britain: 1950–1975* (London: Allen and Unwin).
Younghusband, E. (1981), *The Newest Profession: A Short History of Social Work* (Sutton Community Care, IPC Business Press).

1 *Women and oppression: race, class and gender*

Lesley Day

Introduction

Any consideration of the experiences of women as social work clients and workers should not proceed without examining the intersections between racial, class and gender oppression. The debate within social work about these different forms of oppression has a somewhat chequered history. The radical social work movement, informed by a Marxist analysis, introduced class as a central organizing concept; then feminism raised gender as a crucial issue; and most recently, anti-racist activists have put race and racism on the agenda of social work practice. However, it has not necessarily been the case that the relations between class, gender and race have been clearly identified, or how these relations affect women's lives. The objective of this chapter is not directly to examine this social work literature, but to focus upon feminist ideas and the black feminist critique as a way of enhancing our understanding of how class and race affect the experiences of women.

Women and class

The radical social work movement of the 1970s and early 1980s was largely gender blind (see for example Bailey and Brake 1975; Bolger *et al.* 1981; Jones 1983). In their concern to put an analysis of class and class inequalities on to the agenda for practitioners, these mostly male writers ignored issues of institutionalized sexism and gender inequalities. At the same time, however, the women's movement has been criticized both from within and without for being a middle-class movement. This criticism takes a number of different forms, but one common objection is that it has paid insufficient attention to the specific experiences and interests of working-class women, and has thus contributed to the failure to engage with them personally and politically (Mitchell 1986; Wilson 1989). This class blindness, argues Mitchell, was not surprising given that many feminists were middle class. Hence the women's movement tended to project the particular concerns of middle-class women as the universal interests of all classes of women. As we shall see, it also treated white women's experiences as if they were universal.

The women's movement embodied different analyses of women's oppression. Radical feminists argued that the unequal and disadvantaged position of women flowed fundamentally from the exercise of male power; they insisted on patriarchy as the central organizing category. Thus, as Hartmann points out, some radical feminists argued that the 'original and basic class division is between the sexes' (Hartmann 1981: 13). However, defining women as a class raises difficult theoretical and political issues. Women have different – indeed antagonistic – class interests, and thus their experiences and perceptions of their position vary; as a result working-class women confronted the women's movement about its classism (Wilson 1989). Black women have also challenged the radical feminist analysis, arguing for recognition of the specificity of their experiences as black women living in a racist society.

A different kind of criticism has come from Erik Olin Wright, who has argued that women cannot be conceived of as a class, and that class domination is not the same as oppression. Like men, women own what he terms different types and amounts of productive assets, and thus occupy different positions within the social relations of production. Women may, therefore, exploit one another. Wright rejects the radical feminist analysis:

> This assimilation of women's oppression to class has had the effect both of obscuring the specificity of the oppression of women, and of reducing the theoretical coherence of the concept of class. A more constructive strategy is to examine the relationship between class and gender mechanisms of oppression to try to elaborate a dynamic theory of their interaction and the conditions for the transformation of each of them (Wright 1978: 130).

Wright's approach has much in common with the socialist feminist perspective. Socialist feminism insists on the need for historical specificity about the relationship between the nature of women's oppression and the economic and social organization of society (Barrett 1980; Hartmann 1981). The exploitation of women's labour, paid and unpaid, has to be understood within the context of capitalist society. However, many socialist feminists also take it as axiomatic that gender relations are not solely the effect of capitalism. Patriarchal relations existed before capitalism and 'as far as we can tell, a socialist revolution would not of itself abolish these' (Barrett 1980: 9). Thus, we have to attempt to identify the manner in which patriarchy has become embedded in, and partially constructed by, capitalism.

Within this theoretical framework, the organization of the domestic household is regarded as being closely connected with the nature of paid work undertaken by women in the labour market. Women occupy a position within the sexual division of labour in which they have always been the primary carers for children and other dependent adults. Men are seen as the primary breadwinners upon whom women and children are assumed to be financially dependent, although for many working-class households the notion of the family wage has always been an unattainable ideal: staying above the poverty line still necessitates a two-wage household (Low Pay Unit 1989). This sexual division of labour has weakened women's position in paid employment and has often restricted them to low-paid, insecure and part-time work (Lonsdale 1985; Pascall 1986).

However, while the socialist feminist analysis directed particular attention to the social and economic position of working-class women, and thus to the way the sexual division of labour was mediated by class, the women's movement as a whole never pushed these issues to the forefront of the debate. Looking back over the past twenty years from 1986, Mitchell has argued that the women's movement went through two stages. Firstly, it wanted to 'right the wrongs' experienced by women, by arguing for equal pay and employment opportunities and altering the way in which women's sexuality was viewed. Secondly, it aimed to question and reverse men's views of women as simply mothers and carers. This work needed to be revalued, but it was also something men needed to share. Equality with men, both in paid employment and in the household, was the aim. Mitchell points out, however, that: 'In recognising on paper the class and race distinctions of women but being unable, by definition, to make them the focal thrust of our movement, we contributed to an ideology that temporarily homogenised social classes' (Mitchell 1986: 45).

The women's movement gave insufficient attention to the meaning of the 'double shift' for working-class women. It failed to examine the particular consequences of its perspectives for the lives of working-class women. A woman's experience of the double shift has a different meaning depending on the kind of paid work she does, the wage she receives, the status attached to this work as a female employee, the physical environments in which these different forms of labour take place, and the resources she has to manage and carry out the organization of the domestic household and child care. Some women are able to gain or retain their professional position within the labour market, and thus receive a greater economic reward despite remaining responsible for the organization of the domestic household and child care.[1] Some women may have the choice to be able to pay for other women to take responsibility for some of the domestic labour as well as the manner in which this occurs; they can hire a nanny rather than a childminder, a housekeeper rather than a part-time cleaner. This is not to ignore the fact that all women, directly or indirectly, are primarily responsible for domestic labour and child care, or that the costs of becoming a mother are high in any social class (Moss 1989). It is important to recognize, however, that women's experiences of the sexual division of labour are mediated by their class position.

If the class position of women is seen as central to understanding their everyday lives and experiences, then it follows that we have to take account of how their gendered experiences of the welfare state, and particularly social work, are mediated and affected by living in a class-divided society. Women are much more likely than men to experience social work intervention, because of their roles as mothers, wives, and carers of other dependants (Brook and Davis 1985). The experiences of working-class women make it much more likely that they will seek help from the personal social services, whether because of housing or financial difficulties, or because these or other circumstances have affected their own personal and emotional lives or those of other members of their family. Intervention in their lives may also occur even when it is not sought by them; for example, someone for whom they are thought to be responsible may be deemed to be at risk either physically, emotionally or mentally, and considered to be in need of protection.

As we are, therefore, primarily concerned with working-class women's experiences of social work intervention, we have to understand how sexism and classism can affect the way in which their predicament and experiences are analysed and responded to. Certainly, a radical analysis of the welfare state (Gough 1979) has encouraged a more sophisticated understanding of the contradictory experiences of working-class people who become the recipients of welfare and social work. Yet, this analysis has remained largely gender blind, and has ignored the fact that a working-class woman's experiences of the welfare state are different from those of a working-class man (Williams 1987). The feminist critique of welfare has demonstrated that the welfare state supports and reinforces patriarchal relations, thus confirming the primary responsibilities of women as domestic unpaid workers and child rearers (Wilson 1977). In the late 1970s, however, class and gender analyses of the effects of the welfare state tended to be relatively discrete, and this separation was reflected in the radical social work and feminist social work literature, the former taking class as central, the latter gender.[2]

Clearly both a class and gender analysis are needed if we are to make sense of the specific experiences of working-class female social work clients. We must also take account, however, of the question of race.

Race and gender: the black feminist critique

Our discussion of gender and class has highlighted the fact that feminist theory, politics and practice are riven with difference and difficulty. The absence of any single body of thought or practice has become even more apparent with the emergence of the black feminist critique. Over the last decade, black women have criticized consistently both the women's movement and feminism for their racism, and thus have alerted us to the silence on issues of race and racism in the feminist social work debate up until very recently.[3]

Black feminists contend that women within the women's movement have taken action, written and spoken about their experiences and those of other women from an almost wholly white (and middle-class) perspective. They have, therefore, been subject to racist bias, and much of the literature has rendered black women's lives, and the specificity of their experiences, invisible. In addition, they argue that black women's experiences cannot be simply 'added in' to feminist analysis to overcome their invisibility (Carby 1982; Ramazanoglu 1986). Rather, they insist that feminist theory must be transformed radically to take account of the institutional racism in British society, and thus the inequalities of power and resources which exist between white and black people (Bhavnani 1986). This means that we have to examine, for example, the power relationships between black and white women, white women and black men, and black women and black men. As Bhavnani and Coulson have argued, 'White women entering these debates must acknowledge the material basis of their power in relation to black people, male and female' (Bhavnani and Coulson 1986: 82).

The analysis of racism fundamentally challenges some of the key concepts and assumptions of mainstream feminist thought (Carby 1982). How can we understand, for example, the position of black men as opposed to white men within the hierarchy of patriarchy? Are the concepts of sisterhood and commonality still valid? What are the parallels, if any, between racial and sexual oppression?

Black women writers have emphasized that, in a racist society, their central concern is racial oppression and the gender specificity of racism. Whether they are middle class or working class, black women experience racism. The analysis of racism centres around an understanding of the shared history of oppression experienced by black people from the Asian subcontinent, Africa and the Caribbean as a result of colonialism, and the ways in which the British state and its institutions continue to reproduce racist oppression. The use of the term black signifies the commonality of black people's oppression (Mama 1984). The Organisation of Women of Asian and African Descent emphasized that black women share common 'historical experiences as victims of colonization, and that their present experiences as second class citizens in a racist society create firm bonds between them' (cited in Amos and Parmar 1981: 131).

For anti-racist activists the key concepts are race and racism, and not ethnicity and ethnocentrism. They recognize the specific and different cultural experiences and histories of black women and men, but insist that to become preoccupied with, or to privilege, questions of ethnicity, is to introduce a source of potential ideological and political danger. Sivanandan has pointed out that a celebration of ethnicity and ethnic differences can lead to divisions within the black community, thus detracting from the common fight against racial oppression (Sivanandan 1985).

Furthermore, Carby argues that focusing upon ethnicity and ethnic differences can itself be racist, or at least legitimize racism, because this approach distracts us from a concern with the effects of racism on black women's lives (Carby 1982). Instead, the day-to-day problems facing black women are interpreted as the result of cultural differences, or even, at worst, cultural inferiority. Where cultural differences are reinterpreted as deficits, black women as mothers may be identified as the bearers and transmitters of these deficits. The twists and turns of this approach mean that black women are open to blame whatever they do, and racist stereotypes about their lives and their relationships with men and their children are reaffirmed.

In defence of ethnicity, however, other feminist writers have argued that the category 'black women' excludes many women who are neither British nor black, but who share similar experiences of immigration and discrimination (Anthias and Yuval-Davies 1983). Clearly, women from different ethnic groups suffer the effects of immigration controls and difficulties in the labour market, yet the ethno-centrism of the women's movement has meant that their specific experiences and needs have been largely ignored. Without denying the validity of these experiences, however, black activists reply that these do not justify conflating racism and ethnicity. 'Discarding racism as an unhelpful concept and the black/white distinction as unsatisfactory would neither eradicate racism, nor would it be acceptable to black women' (Kazi 1986:89).

Carby insists that feminist theories cannot be sufficiently transformed by incorporating more knowledge of the diversity of cultures of black women and thus 'blackening' feminist theory. Rather the central tool of analysis has to be racism, and its effects upon black women's lives.

Patriarchy – a white concept?

There is a wide range of criticisms of feminist theory in terms of its race blindness and racism. One of the fundamental challenges the black feminist movement has made is in its analysis of patriarchal power relationships between black men and black women. It has challenged the radical feminist position that patriarchal power is a transhistorical phenomenon and that the oppression of women by (all) men is the most fundamental and intractable form of oppression (Joseph 1981; Carby 1982; Amos and Parmar 1984).

For example, we gain a different perspective on roles within the family and women's relationships with members of their households if we consider the accounts of, and analyses by, Asian women (Trivedi 1984; Ahmed 1986; Brah 1987). Colonization was legitimated by the ideology that Britain was a liberalizing force, and one aspect of this was the view that women in Asian families were passive and subordinate to their husbands. As Brah points out, however, while it was the case that the British did 'liberalize the law on some issues, on others their policies had the effect of either reinforcing existing gender inequality or creating a new form which was as, if not more, oppressive to women' (Brah 1987: 44). The contemporary ideological construction of Asian women's lives, although specific to present day socio-economic conditions, draws upon this colonial past. We know, however, that Asian women are challenging these definitions of themselves, and coming together both within specific organizations and within the more private domain of home and community, to discuss the shape and future of their lives (Trivedi 1984; Brah 1987).

For white women the message is clear. Firstly, we should not collude with or give credence to racist stereotypes of the passive and submissive Asian woman, but recognize the difficulties that Asian women face in confronting sexist practices and racial oppression. Secondly, it is a racist assumption on the part of white women to assume that Asian women are in a fundamentally different position from white women and need to be liberated from these oppressive structures. The example sometimes cited by white women is arranged marriages, which seem to be more oppressive than marriage customs in white western cultures. However, we should recognize not only that the amount of choice available to Asian girls varies considerably within the Asian community, but also that the choice of marriage partner of many white girls, although set within the context of romantic love, is also subject to parental supervision and class boundaries (Amos and Parmar 1981). Thus, we should guard against assuming that certain cultural practices are self-evidently more oppressive than others. This can lead to denial of the constructive nature of parental and other familial relationships within the Asian community. Amos and Parmar make their position clear: 'We demand the right to choose and struggle around the issue of family oppression ourselves within our own communities, without state intervention and without white feminists making judgements as to the oppressive nature of arranged marriages' (Amos and Parmar 1984: 15).

Other black women writers (Joseph 1981; Carby 1982) reject the assumption that the dominance of black males can be equated with white male dominance. Carby argues that to understand black women's lives and their family structures we have to examine how colonization shaped and affected the sex/gender systems of a society, and how these are changed by migration (Carby 1982). Similarly, we need to understand the ways in which imperialism may have reinforced and distorted oppressive relations within families, as well as destroying some of their more non-oppressive and communal relations. In some instances this may lead to men gaining more power *vis-à-vis* children and women, in others less (Caulfield 1974).

For the Afro-Caribbean community, slavery fundamentally affected the power relationships between black women and men. Speaking of slavery in America, Joseph argues that the black male was 'disallowed a superior position in relation to the black female' (Joseph 1981: 99). Family networks were the primary mechanisms through which 'slave women and men devised organisational forms for the survival of the young, and maintained cultural patterns of resistance to, and rebellion against, the coloniser' (Caulfield 1974: 72). Cooperative mechanisms for looking after and bringing up children, sharing work and so on, were means of defence and resistance. Migration affects these family structures. However, strong female networks, and the fact that women are likely to occupy key positions in the development of strategies to resist and fight against institutionalized racism in this society, remain an important feature of black women's lives (Carby 1982).

Thus, the sexism of black males and their power *vis-à-vis* black women is not ignored (Hooks 1982; 1984; Marable 1983). The black women's movement simply insists that these problems cannot be understood or tackled in the same way as the sexism and power of white men. Some black women identify their position as one where they 'struggle together with black men against racism, while we also struggle with black men, about sexism' (Carby 1982: 213).

Race, class and gender

A number of points follow from the theoretical and political debates about race, class and gender. Firstly, the parallels between racism and sexism, as different forms of oppression, have to be treated with caution. They may be similarly constructed ideologically in that the 'explanation' for unequal treatment is based upon arguments of natural or biological differences and inferiorities. However, we have to recognize that although both are socially constructed, gender denotes the socially constructed differences which have been built upon the anatomical differences between men and women, whereas race is a socially constructed category which has no basis in anatomy or biology (Barrett and McIntosh 1985). The form of analysis and the institutions to be analysed differ when considering racism and sexism (Carby 1982).

Secondly, it is evident that if we are to gain any kind of real understanding of women's lives, the intersections between racial, class and gender oppression have to be recognized. Bourne reminds us that if we assert the commonality of women's experiences, we ignore the complexity of their lives and in 'claiming to liberate women from their biological determinism' we have to take care not to 'deny women an existence outside that determined by their sex' (Bourne 1983: 19). Thus, class position and race reconstruct women's gendered experiences in a class divided and racist society.

Women as clients: motherhood and family life

Since motherhood and women's pivotal position in the family make it more likely that they, rather than men, will become social work clients, there are many common elements in the predicament of women as clients. However, we must consider also the ways in which these gendered experiences are mediated by class and race, and specifically how black and working-class women are treated by social workers and their agencies.

Motherhood

The social construction of motherhood, and the ways in which the state views women as mothers, have been subjected to considerable feminist analyses (Badinter 1981; Antonis 1981; David 1985; 1986). While a positive value is conferred on women who are mothers, and indeed if you are married it is thought to be unnatural not to want to be a mother (MacIntyre 1976), women receive little support as mothers, as it is assumed that they are dependent upon a man.

Notions of what makes a good mother are very often middle class, thus making working-class women at greater risk of intervention by the welfare state (David 1985). The material circumstances of some women and their double shift also make taking care of children an extremely difficult and tiring job, which the state only comes to recognize when they fail to achieve certain standards. Working-class women are in a contradictory position. They are subject to the dominant ideology that their primary role is to mother, but their economic circumstances, with or without a partner, often make it imperative for them to seek paid work. The economy recognizes their value and usefulness in certain kinds of occupations but also assigns them predominantly to the secondary labour market.

The social construction of motherhood in relation to black women is far more contradictory. For her the positive value attached to being a mother is contradicted, not simply because she is black and is therefore seen as 'inferior' from a racist viewpoint, but also because she may be viewed as the producer of more black people, and thus perceived as a threat (Williams 1987). Furthermore, the exploitation of black women's labour in paid employment takes a different and racialized form. Irrespective of their position as mothers, women from the Caribbean were primarily seen as a useful reserve army of labour by British capital. Thus: 'Rather than a concern to protect or preserve the black family in Britain, the state reproduced common sense notions of its inherent pathology: black women were seen to fail as mothers precisely because of their position as workers' (Carby 1982: 219). However, it is Afro-Caribbean rather than Asian women who are subject to this form of racism. The stereotypical but mythical view that the Asian woman very rarely works outside the home may have protected her, by some kind of cruel logic, from this particular kind of criticism about her role as a mother.[4]

For working-class white and black women then, undertaking two jobs, paid employment and caring for children, is a common experience. Thus, to understand women's experiences of mothering we also have to take account of the kind of paid work that they do. Feminist analyses have alerted us to the fact that the position of women in the labour market is structured by the ideology of femininity and domesticity; paid work is viewed as secondary to women's primary child care responsibilities, and jobs thought suitable for women draw upon and reproduce appropriate 'feminine' attributes. However, a woman's class position also affects the kind of paid work she can find and be thought suitable for; and for black women their position in the labour market is racialized. For example, Asian women are more commonly found in low-paid, unskilled and non-unionized occupations; even in sectors of the economy where women predominate, Asian women are to be found doing the lowest grade work (Brah 1987).

Both working-class white and black women are vulnerable to state intervention should they fail to be proper mothers, and their ability to mother may also be questioned because they are in paid work. It may also be that the status of their employment negatively reflects upon their skills as a mother. By contrast, a woman in a professional job may be positively evaluated, as the status of her employment is taken as evidence of her ability to mother, and also to find appropriate substitute care for her children. Thus, perceptions of mothering are both class-based and racist. For example, there is the stereotypical notion of the strong, working-class mother who is thought to be a 'good manager' and able to cope with her paid work and domestic responsibilities. However, recognition of her needs and the limit to her coping capacity may be rendered invisible. On the other hand, there is the image of the mother in what used to be termed the 'rough' as opposed to the 'respectable' working-class household. She may be seen as either unable to manage both jobs adequately, or to be deficient as a mother, whether she is in paid employment or not.

Black women's mothering is scrutinized in different ways. For example, there is little understanding of the central role of the mother in Afro-Caribbean families and the value placed upon children. In addition, the absence or marginal position of the black male is either misunderstood or exaggerated (see Bryan in this volume). Furthermore, the impact of racism on a black woman's life and her struggle to care for her children in the way that she would like within her family or community network may be downgraded or dimly understood. Stereotypes of the ever-strong, coping Afro-Caribbean mother may be unquestioningly accepted.

For women of Asian origin, their mothering may be viewed differently again – but still stereotypically. Brah argues that much contemporary writing presents Asian women as 'docile and passive victims of archaic traditional customs and practices, and of domineering Asian men' (Brah 1987: 44). Thus, women may be viewed as being oppressed by their role as mothers, suffocated by domesticity and lacking independence. This perspective ignores the experiences of Asian women as mothers and paid workers, living in a racist society.

A structural analysis of the experiences of motherhood which takes account of the effects of class and race is essential if mothering by white working-class and black women is not to be pathologized. In a different vein, Channer and Parton argue that social workers should guard against a cultural relativism that prevents them from intervening against child abuse in black families, because they accept black families' parenting performances unhesitatingly as culturally different but valid (Channer and Parton 1990). Rather, the impact of racial, sexual and class inequalities, as well as the particular emotional and individual difficulties which a woman is experiencing, have to form the basis of any analysis of mothering. Feminist analyses have alerted us to the need to confirm the difficulties which motherhood causes for women, as well as recognizing their strength in this role (Hale 1983; Hudson 1985). Sexist assumptions about mothering have to be questioned, but so do racist and class-based ones.

Family life

An analysis of women's experiences of family life, mediated by class and race, and the state's relationship to the institution of the family, is central to a social worker's ability to comprehend the complexity of women's lives. Barrett and McIntosh have argued that the family is oppressive to women, that it is an 'anti-social' institution (Barrett and McIntosh 1982). The monogamous nuclear family form promotes individualistic rather than social or collective values, and its privatized nature excludes those outside it. They further argue that the welfare state privileges this form of family, thus confirming the dependency of women on men within the household, and penalizing those women who do not live within it.

This analysis has been criticized as partial and racist (Bhavnani and Coulson 1986). Firstly, black women writers have questioned whether the black family can be conceptualized as anti-social. Secondly, they argue that insufficient attention has been paid to the specificity of black women's experiences of the welfare state. These two arguments are linked in that the black family is seen to be an important source of support and resistance against racism, and particularly the institutional racism of the welfare state and its agencies.

The argument that black families cannot be conceived of as anti-social is a complex and contradictory one. Black feminists point to black women's positive experiences of family life, where alliances and relationships are forged on the basis of a common recognition of, and resistance to, racism. This does not mean that they ignore the sexism of black men or that they fail to recognize the fact that the ideology of mother/wife roles is oppressive to black women as well as white women (Amos and Parmar 1984). What they question is the view that black women are more oppressed in the family than white women. In a study of Asian and white adolescent girls and boys and their parents, Brah concluded that views about the sexual division of labour were similar and that both Asian and white women's views 'embodied elements of collusion, resistance and opposition' (Brah 1987: 47). Black women are confronting issues of concern to them that arise out of their familial and household relationships. For example, black women are assessing their experiences of male violence and demanding the services which will best serve their needs. However, they are having to fight both racism and sexism in that they also have to confront the racist stereotypes of white people about their sexuality, their femininity and their mothering (Trivedi 1984; Ahmed 1986). Bhavnani and Coulson sum up black women's experiences of the family:

> Whatever inequalities exist in such [black] households, they are also clearly sites of support for their members. In saying this, we are recognizing that black women may have significant issues to face within black households (Bhavnani and Coulson 1986: 88).

Several authorities have documented the effects of institutional racism in housing, social security, education, health and the personal social services (for example Gordon and Newnham 1985; Troyna 1987; Ginsburg 1989). The construction and operation of immigration laws shows clearly how the state upholds the integrity and sanctity of only certain kinds of families – white ones. Similarly, in the child care system, the over-representation of black children in care and the under-recruitment of black foster parents (Ahmed, Cheetham and Small 1986) suggest that the black family is treated differently. The paradox is, however, that the sanctity of the black family, and particularly Asian families, may be invoked when assumptions are made by social welfare agencies that these households are self-supporting. In addition, women's needs as carers of dependent members of their families are likely to remain ignored (Williams 1987).

Other feminists have pointed out that for white working-class women too, experiences of family life are contradictory. Despite their thesis that the nuclear family is anti-social, Barrett and McIntosh themselves recognize that marriage is not only popular, but that it can meet real emotional and psychological needs (Barrett and McIntosh 1982). Jane Humphries goes much further, arguing that the family as benefited working-class men and women, providing a base for resistance against the instrusions of the welfare state. It is important to consider, therefore, whether a parallel argument to the one about the black family and its fight against racism can be made in relation to the working-class family (Humphries 1977). A contemporary example of the strength of the working-class family was provided by the 1984–5 miners' strike in Britain. Miners' wives fought with and supported their men in the strike, while at the same time gaining strength as women together. We have to take account of the fact, therefore, that working-class women and men share class experiences and common perceptions of their position in society, and thus form alliances in opposition to external threats to their family life.

It is not only black families that may be seen in a negative or discriminatory way. Any family structure which does not conform to the idealized notion of the nuclear family may be penalized and treated differently by the welfare state. Concerns about the single mother and her dependency upon the state rather than a man have led government ministers to propose policy changes which would discourage single parents and emphasize the financial responsibilities of fathers for their children.

If we are to understand the 'anti-social' nature of women's experiences of family life, an analysis which takes account of class and race is of paramount importance. This does not detract from, but enhances any analysis and comprehension of the oppression that women experience in the family. Furthermore, Ahmed has argued that it is necessary to be sensitive to cultural differences in family relationships, and not to employ an over-simplified analysis which relies on negative stereotypes, and which can reconstruct cultural differences as deficits (Ahmed 1986). However, cultural awareness should not be at the expense of employing other analyses of the lives of black women and their families. As Ahmed points out:

> The argument is not against better cultural understanding but against an over-reliance on cultural explanations which distract attention both from significant emotional factors as well as structural factors, such as class and race (Ahmed 1986: 140).

Although this argument applies to black women, and specifically to social work clients, it can also be employed in relation to white working-class women, who may also be subject to cultural misconceptions, and the nature of their gendered experiences misunderstood and oversimplified.

Women social workers

Class and race are not only crucial to our understanding of the lives of female social work clients, but also to the position and working experience of the social worker, and her relationship with her clients. It is now well-documented that women predominate at the basic grade level of social work (Popplestone 1980; Howe 1986; Walby 1987). As we move up the management hierarchy, however, women become less and less visible. In addition, social work has always been class divided. From its earliest days in the late nineteenth century, social work was thought of as a suitable occupation for middle-class women, who could dispense their caring skills to poor working-class women and assist them to perform their domestic and child care responsibilities more effectively (Brook and Davis 1985). Residential work, which was thought to require less skill, was more often undertaken by working-class women. These class divisions still exist; women from working-class origins are more evident in what are often perceived to be the less prestigious areas of social work, those associated with basic caring (for example, day care of children under five, and residential work). Working-class women also predominate on social work training courses such as the Certificate in Social Services, which are often perceived by students as having lower status.

The class position of (women) social workers has been the subject of much debate. There is considerable disagreement among, for example, Marxist writers, about the class position of what are referred to as 'non-productive state workers'. For example, Erik Olin Wright suggests that basic grade social workers (and probably lower-level managers) occupy 'contradictory class locations', as neither part of the bourgeoisie nor the working class (Wright 1978). They do not have control over the creation of state social policies or the production of ideology; rather, they execute the policies of the state and disseminate its ideology. However, Wright also points out that because of their contradictory position, social workers have contradictory class interests and can, therefore, 'potentially be organised into more than one class capacity' (Wright 1978: 108). Put another way, we need to distinguish between state power and the position of social workers. Other analyses of the state have exposed its bourgeois, racist and sexist nature (Williams 1989). While the female social worker can be understood as the bearer or victim of these forms of oppression, she also has some capacity – albeit limited – to resist these aspects of state domination (London Edinburgh Weekend Return Group 1979; Hudson 1985; Ahmed, Cheetham and Small 1986).

This analytic framework enables us to consider a number of issues in relation to the employment of black women social workers. Firstly, the positions they occupy in social work are racialized, as in other occupations (Phizacklea 1983). Black women may be perceived as being more suitable for some social work tasks and jobs than others. Carby has argued, for example, that black women have been seen as especially suitable for working as nurses or care assistants (Carby 1982); hence black women are found in the lowest status occupations. We also find black women employed predominantly in residential care of the elderly and as care assistants in children's homes. They are not so visible in the more prestigious areas such as family work, which demand therapeutic intervention in families.

Secondly, Stubbs has pointed to the danger that more black (women) social workers may be employed in the personal social services as a way of dealing with the needs of black clients rather than as a move towards eliminating discriminatory employment practices in social services departments and voluntary organizations (Stubbs 1985). Furthermore, black women workers may be seen as the 'cultural experts . . . without being given any real opportunity to question the assumptions which are at the heart of the management of particular cases' (Stubbs 1985: 18). Nor should the employment of black women social workers be seen as the solution to the culturally racist practices of some white workers. Black social workers are resisting these definitions of their employment and challenging the institutionalized racism of the personal social services. However, as Stubbs points out, it is a constant battle to resist being 'forced into a model of the good black social worker' who fits unquestioningly into the existing racist structures (Stubbs 1985: 17).

A similar argument can be made in relation to the white female social worker. We have documented how feminism has been slow to articulate the specific experiences of black and working-class women. In addition, mainstream feminist ideas have remained largely invisible and marginalized on social work courses (see Carter, Everitt and Hudson in this volume). It is no surprise that many women workers play out the model of the 'good female social worker', who does not threaten (or at worst reproduces) the sexist-based structures in which she operates.

As we see from other chapters in this book, and from the growing literature on feminist social work practice (for example Hanmer and Statham 1988), working in an anti-sexist way is surrounded with difficulty. However, when race and class are introduced into the equation the issues to be confronted by black and white female social workers become even more complex. If we are to gain a better understanding of how women workers and their female clients encounter each other in the personal social services, what assumptions and judgements they may make about each other, and how the state determines the form that these relationships can take, issues of race, class and gender are pivotal.

Notes

1 Although we should note that parenthood for women can lead to downward occupational mobility (Moss 1989).
2 One of the recent additions to this literature, by Hanmer and Statham, does, however, take account of class issues (Hanmer and Statham 1988).
3 For example, Hanmer and Statham (1988) make some reference to race, and Ahmed, Cheetham and Small (1986) and Dominelli (1988), take race and racism as central, although they are not exclusively concerned with woman-centred practice.
4 Although Asian women came to Great Britain as dependents of male workers, employment data now show that a high proportion of Asian women are in paid employment (Parmar 1982; Barrett and McIntosh 1985; Brah 1987).

References

Ahmed, S. (1986), 'Cultural racism in work with Asian women and girls', in S. Ahmed, J. Cheetham and J. Small (eds), *Social Work with Black Children and their Families* (London: Batsford).
Ahmed, S., Cheetham, J., and Small, J. (eds) (1986), *Social Work with Black Children and their Families* (London: Batsford).
Amos, V., and Parmar, P. (1981), 'Resistances and responses: black girls in Britain', in A. McRobbie and T. McCabe (eds), *Feminism for Girls: An Adventure Story* (London: Routledge and Kegan Paul).
Amos, V., and Parmar, P. (1984), 'Challenging imperial feminism: gender, ethnic and class divisions', *Feminist Review* 15.
Anthias, F., and Yuval-Davis, N. (1983), 'Contextualizing feminism: gender, ethnic and class divisions', *Feminist Review* 15.
Antonis, B. (1981), 'Motherhood and mothering', in The Cambridge Women's Studies Group (eds) *Women in Society* (London: Virago).

Badinter, E. (1981), *The Myth of Motherhood* (London: Souvenir Press).
Bailey, R., and Brake, M. (eds) (1975), *Radical Social Work* (London: Edward Arnold).
Barrett, M. (1980), *Women's Oppression Today* (London: Verso).
Barrett, M., and McIntosh, M. (1982), *The Anti-Social Family* (London: Verso).
Barrett, M., and McIntosh, M. (1985), 'Ethnocentrism and socialist-feminist theory', *Feminist Review* 20.
Beagley, J. (1986), 'Why men manage and women are the workforce', *Community Care Supplement*, 18 September.
Bhavnani, K., and Coulson, M. (1986), 'Transforming socialist-feminism; the challenge of racism', *Feminist Review* 23.
Bolger, S., Corrigan, R., Docking, J., and Frost, N. (1981), *Towards Socialist Welfare Work* (London: Macmillan).
Bourne, J. (1983), 'Towards an anti-racist feminism', *Race and Class*, XXV, 1.

Brah, A. (1987), 'Women of South Asian origin in Britain: issues and concerns', *South Asia Research* 7, 1.
Brook, E., and Davis, A. (eds) (1985), *Women, the Family and Social Work* (London: Tavistock).
Bryan, F., Dadzie, S., and Scafe, S. (1985), *The Heart of the Race: Black Women's Lives in Britain* (London: Virago).

Carby, H. (1982), 'White women listen! black feminism and the boundaries of sisterhood', in Centre for Contemporary Cultural Studies (eds), *The Empire Strikes Back: Race and Racism in 70s Britain* (London: Hutchinson).
Caulfield, M. (1974), 'Imperialism, the family and cultures of resistance', *Socialist Revolution* 20, 4.
Channer, Y., and Parton, N. (1990), 'Racism, cultural relativism and child protection', in The Violence Against Children Study Group (eds), *Taking Child Abuse Seriously: Contemporary Issues in Child Protection Theory and Practice* (London: Unwin Hyman).

David, M. (1985), 'Motherhood and social policy: a matter of education', *Critical Social Policy* 12.
David, M. (1986), 'Morality and maternity: towards a better union than the moral right's family policy', *Critical Social Policy* 16.
Davis, A. (1981), *Women, Race and Class* (London: The Women's Press).
Dominelli, L. (1988), *Anti-Racist Social Work* (London: Macmillan Education).

Finch, J., and Groves, D. (eds) (1983), *A Labour of Love: Women, Work and Caring* (London: Routledge and Kegan Paul).

Ginsburg, N. (1989), 'Institutional racism and local authority housing', *Critical Social Policy* 24.
Gordon, P., and Newnham, A. (1985), *Passports to Benefits: Racism in Social Security* (London: Child Poverty Action Group and the Runnymede Trust).
Gough, I. (1979), *The Political Economy of the Welfare State* (London: Macmillan).

Hale, J. (1983), 'Feminism and social work practice', in B. Jordan and N. Parton (eds), *The Political Dimensions of Social Work* (Oxford: Basil Blackwell).
Hanmer, J., and Statham, D. (1988), *Women and Social Work: Towards a Woman-Centred Practice* (London: Macmillan Education).
Hartmann, H., *et al.* (1981), *The Unhappy Marriage of Marxism and Feminism: Towards a More Progressive Union* in L. Sargent (ed.), *The Unhappy Marriage of Marxism and Feminism, A Debate on Class and Patriarchy* (London: Pluto Press).
Hooks, B. (1982), *Ain't I a Woman: Black Women and Feminism* (London: Pluto Press).
Hooks, B. (1984), *Feminist Theory: From Margin to Center* (Boston: South End Press).

Hooks, B. (1986), 'Sisterhood: political solidarity between women', *Feminist Review* 23.
Howe, D. (1986), 'The segregation of women and their work in the personal social services', *Critical Social Policy* 15.
Hudson, A. (1985), 'Feminism and social work; resistance or dialogue?', *British Journal of Social Work* 15.
Humphries, J. (1977), 'Class struggle and the persistence of the working class family', *Cambridge Journal of Economics* 1, 3.

Jones, C. (1983), *State Social Work and the Working Class* (London: Macmillan).
Joseph, G. (1981), 'The incompatible menage a trois: marxism, feminism, and racism', in L. Sargent (ed.), *The Unhappy Marriage of Marxism and Feminism, A Debate on Class and Patriarchy* (London: Pluto Press).

Kazi, H. (1986), 'The beginning of a debate long due: some observations on ethnocentrism and socialist-feminist theory', *Feminist Review* 22.

Lewis, G., and Parmar, P. (1983), 'Black women's writing', *Race and Class* XXV, 2.
London Edinburgh Weekend Return Group (1979), *In and Against the State* (London: Pluto Press).
Lonsdale, S. (1985), *Work and Inequality* (Harlow: Longman).
Low Pay Unit (1989), *Written Evidence to House of Commons Select Committee on Employment* 26 April, Session 1988/9 (London: Low Pay Unit).

Macintyre, S. (1976), 'Who wants babies? The social construction of instincts' in D. Barker and S. Allan (eds), *Sexual Divisions and Society* (London: Tavistock).
Mama, A. (1984), 'Black women, the economic crisis and the British state', *Feminist Review* 17.
Marable, M. (1983), *How Capitalism Underdeveloped Black America* (Boston: South End Press).
Mitchell, J. (1986), 'Reflections on twenty years of feminism', in J. Mitchell and A. Oakley (eds), *What is Feminism?* (London: Basil Blackwell).
Moss, P. (1989), 'The indirect costs of parenthood: a neglected issue in social policy', *Critical Social Policy* 24.
Murphy, L., and Livingstone, J. (1985), 'Racism and the limits of radical feminism', *Race and Class* XXVI, 4.

Parmar, P. (1982), 'Gender, race and class: Asian women in resistance', in Centre for Contemporary Cultural Studies (eds), *The Empire Strikes Back: Race and Racism in 70s Britain* (London: Hutchinson).
Pascall, G. (1986), *Social Policy: A Feminist Analysis* (London: Tavistock).
Phizacklea, A. (1983), *One Way Ticket; Migration and Female Labour* (London: Routledge and Kegan Paul).
Popplestone, R. (1980), 'Top jobs for women: are the cards stacked against them', *Social Work Today* 12, 4.

Ramazanoglu, C. (1986), 'Ethnocentrism and socialist-feminist theory: a response to Barrett and McIntosh', *Feminist Review* 22.

Sivanandan, A. (1985), 'RAT and the degradation of Black struggle', *Race and Class* XXVI, 4.

Stubbs, P. (1985), 'The employment of Black social workers: from ethnic sensitivity to anti-racism?', *Critical Social Policy* 12.

Trivedi, P. (1984), 'To deny our fullness: Asian women in the making of history', *Feminist Review* 17.

Troyna, B. (ed.) (1987), *Racial Inequality in Education* (London: Tavistock).

Walby, C. (1987), 'Why are so few women working in senior positions?', *Social Work Today*, 16 February.

Williams, F. (1987), 'Racism and the discipline of social policy', *Critical Social Policy* 20.

Williams, F. (1989), *Social Policy: A Critical Introduction* (London: Polity Press).

Wilson, E. (1977), *Women and the Welfare State* (London: Tavistock).

Wilson, E. (1989), 'Feedback', *Critical Social Policy* 24.

Wright, E. (1978), *Class, Crisis and the State* (London: Verso).

2 *Women's psychology and feminist social work practice*

Marilyn Lawrence

Introduction

This chapter discusses some of the important changes which have taken place in our understanding of women's psychology over the last two decades. A deeper and more careful understanding of women's psychological development is essential if social workers are to find a more helpful response to women clients. The psychological welfare of children is inseparable from that of their mothers, and any notion of 'child protection' needs to take account of this. Much of the argument centres around the nature of the mother/daughter relationship, and suggests that women's development has to be understood within a context that is psychologically and emotionally fraught and difficult.

Any explanation that rests upon a particular pattern of social and personal relationships has to address the question of whether or not it is universally applicable, that is, whether or not it can be assumed to cut across different social class and racial groups. To what extent, for example, is the literature on the mother/daughter relationship in contemporary society applicable to black women?

In tackling these questions, I shall draw upon feminist psychoanalytic theories developed in Britain and North America. The most well-known and accessible exponents of these theories are Luise Eichenbaum and Susie Orbach (1983) the founders of the Women's Therapy Centre in London. The Centre has continued to develop its ideas around women's psychological development. The work of Ernst and Maguire (1987) demonstrates the great potential of this kind of theory for understanding a wide range of life situations in which women find themselves.

It is probably true to say that, like most feminist initiatives, the Women's Therapy Centre initially focused on the experience of white women. It is part of the Centre's current project to test out, extend and reframe its ideas in relation to black women's experience, and this chapter is intended as a contribution to that undertaking.

Before considering some of the recent developments in feminist psychology, it is important to look very briefly at the legacy of psychoanalysis itself and to see just what it was that feminists have been left to develop and transform.

One of the most important achievements of the women's liberation movement over the past decade has been the recognition that psychology has been formulated on assumptions which make the experience of men the primary focus of attention, and take no account of the fact that women's experience might be different. This is a particularly serious state of affairs in developmental psychology, which purports to tell us why we have become the way we are. If, at this very fundamental level of explanation, assumptions are made about the roles of women and men and the relationships between them, then not only are the conclusions flawed, but we can become trapped in a set of misunderstandings which have implications for the way we understand adult women and men.

The legacy of psychoanalysis

The most interesting recent developments in our understanding of women's psychology have taken place within psychoanalytic thinking. Psychoanalysis has never been quite sure of its ground on women. Feminists have rightly criticized Freud for the supreme place he gave to biology and the body, while all but ignoring social reality. However, it has to be said in his defence, that Freud was not content with his own formulations on female sexuality and recognized that much work remained to be done (Freud 1964). Within the first generation of psychoanalysts, women analysts took up the challenge. Karen Horney and Clara Thompson, amongst others, suggested that Freud's work lacked sufficient understanding of the social position of women and the effect of this on their emotional development. Baker Miller has collected together some of the most interesting papers written by these early women psychoanalysts (Baker Miller 1973).

The debates and controversies surrounding women have continued within the psychoanalytic establishment up to the present day. Contemporary psychoanalysts Juliet Mitchell (1975), Janine Chasseguet-Smirgel (1985) and Christiane Olivier (1989) have offered readings of Freud which enrich and extend the psychoanalytical perspective on women's psychology.

The school of psychoanalysis which probably lends itself best to an understanding of the importance of gender and race as key developmental issues is the British tradition often known as object relations theory. The chief exponents of this are Fairbairn, Guntrip and the very influential D. W. Winnicott.[1] These psychoanalysts moved away from the narrow confines of the triad of mother/father/child as the crucible in which development takes place, and focused instead on the much earlier stages of development in which the baby and mother (or caretaker) are the only important figures. The object relations theorists are also part of a tradition which places special emphasis on the real and unique experience of each individual. This tradition allows that any kind of deprivation or impingement on development can have real effects. This is obviously crucial in any account of the development of a group disadvantaged by gender, class or race. Much of the theoretical work of the Women's Therapy Centre takes this psychoanalytical position as a starting point. It is clear however that even within the 'feminist psychoanalytic tradition', there is no single common interpretation of gender. The wide range of assessments of the treatment of gender both in traditional psychoanalysis and in some of the later contributions are well documented and discussed by Vivien Barr (1987). Pearson *et al.*, in the introduction to *Social Work and the Legacy of Freud* (1988) offer an interesting and very useful overview of developments within psychoanalysis around the issue of women's psychology.

The feminist psychoanalytic perspective

I shall now summarize some of the main formulations of feminist psychoanalytic thinking which I consider to be useful and relevant to certain aspects of social work practice – child care practice in particular.

The first and perhaps most fundamental shift in feminist understanding of women's psychology lies in the recognition that it is subordinate psychology. Jean Baker Miller suggests that women, having no power in their own right, learn – like all subordinate groups – that they can only achieve influence via the superordinate group, i.e. men (Baker Miller 1976). This means that women's concerns are centred on pleasing and affiliation with others rather than on meeting their own needs and asserting their own views. Women experience their very survival as depending upon their ability to please. Throughout her work, Baker Miller draws parallels between the psychic experience of women under patriarchy and that of black people under racism. While this parallel may be controversial, and perhaps inadequate, it points the way to a new understanding of the psychology of oppression.

While this takes us some way towards a radical rethinking of the psychology of women, it begs a number of questions in relation to the experience of black women. The point that Baker Miller is making is that in an institutionally racist society, white people, both women and men, have power over black people, who are the subordinate group. If however, we understand the superordinate group as white men, rather than all men, we might consider the experience of black women living in a white patriarchal and racist society to be quite different from that of white women. One of the key issues is the relationship and proximity of black and white women to white men. The lack of power of black men in British society may suggest that the direct experience of gender oppression for black women may be different from that of white women in very specific ways.

According to Baker Miller, certain aspects of human experience have been recognized, labelled as 'feminine' and then devalued. In particular, caring, intuition, being in touch with feelings and personal creativity are human attributes with which women have been credited, but which have then been devalued and disowned by the dominant group. Baker Miller's great achievement is that she goes on to acknowledge that psychoanalysis deals with precisely these issues:

> What has psychoanalysis really been dealing with? First, Freud focused on bodily, sexual and childish experience and said that these are of determining but hidden importance. More recent psychoanalytic theory tends to emphasize the deeper issues of feelings of vulnerability, weakness, helplessness, dependency, and the basic emotional connections between an individual and other people. That is, psychoanalysis has in a very large sense been engaged in bringing about the acknowledgement of these crucial realms of the human experience. It has done this, I think, without recognizing that these areas of experience have been kept out of people's conscious awareness by virtue of their being so heavily dissociated from men and so heavily associated with women. It is not that men, like all people, do not have experience in these areas. As psychoanalysis has been engaged in pointing out, these are most significant human experiences. Indeed, they involve the necessities of human experience. One might even say that we came to 'need' psychoanalysis precisely because certain essential parts of men's experience have been very problematic, and therefore were unacknowledged, unexplored and denied (Baker Miller 1976: 23).

Here we have a clear statement not only that women and men inhabit very different psychic worlds, but that the inner world of women consists of that which men cannot bear. Baker Miller goes as far as to suggest that psychoanalysis may be an attempt at best to repair the split, at least to make women's experience manageable for men.

Eichenbaum and Orbach (1983) begin their analysis of the essential difference between women and men far back in the mother/daughter relationship, before the father becomes an important figure in the constellation. (The term 'mother' here really stands for caretaker, who might well be a grandmother or an older sister. It is however, almost invariably a woman.) For them, the crucial issue is that the mother and the baby girl share a common gender identity. They do not romanticize this relationship, but rather stress its essential difficulty. Under patriarchy, it is the task of the mother to induct her daughter into the role of second-class citizen. She may not do this in overt ways, but rather through the detail of the relationship she sets up. Like herself, her daughter must orientate herself towards meeting the needs of others. She must learn from her mother to be a carer and not expect to be cared for in any but the most superficial sense. As a woman who has only partially had her own emotional needs met, she encourages her daughter not to expect too much.

We can see this pattern reflected in the day-to-day interaction within families. While the small boy may be empowered and even encouraged to express his own needs and desires, the little girl is likely to be cautioned about the effect this may have on others. 'I know how you feel, but you know it will upset him. Why don't you let him have it? After all he doesn't understand things as well as you do.' The little girl learns that by not asserting herself, by not demanding what she wants, she will reap a greater reward. She can maintain her closeness with her mother by becoming like her mother – a carer – someone for others, not someone for herself.

For many mothers, the sight of an emotionally needy baby girl sets up an unbearable identification with the needy baby girl she carries inside herself. Women often report that on the sight of their new-born baby girls, they felt they saw themselves, there in the cot. While as women we all try to meet our children's needs out of the deep well of our own unmet needs, we have to acknowledge that this is impossible. Try as we may, it is our daughters who all too often suffer our unconscious inability to give what we have not got. For sons, mothers at least have the advantage of difference and a ready-made separation. He is different, the 'other', and thus the mother can give herself time and space to get to know him, understand him and interpret his needs. We have a much less easy relationship with our daughters, who all too often seem like an extension of ourselves, holding our own unmet needs up into the light and filling us with envy and anger.

As we grow up, the daughters of mothers who can neither fully nurture us nor really let us go, women often have a sense of unmet, never-to-be-met need. Many women feel tied and bound to their mothers in a way which doesn't satisfy either of them. We have a sense of our own need, but no way of expressing that need and certainly no sense of how it might be met. We feel beached, like whales washed up on the tide, suspended, stranded with our needs which we feel ashamed to show to others and even to acknowledge to ourselves.

Here again we have to ask a question about the experience of black women in terms of the dynamics of the mother/daughter relationship. Given the rather different nature of the gender oppression suffered by black women in a white patriarchal society, we might suppose that the black mother has the dual job of preparing her daughter for her role in a society which will oppress her both for being a woman and being black. The specific nature of the mother's own oppression, and her accommodation to it will thus be unconsciously re-experienced and transmitted to the baby girl.

To want to be cared for can feel as if we are being very demanding, unreasonable, difficult. Yet as women, we know we must be ready to take 24-hour responsibility for others. This is a situation which might be expected to call forth anger and frustration from women. But, unlike men, women are not encouraged to express negative emotions. Anger, rage and hatred – all perfectly normal human emotions – are forbidden for women. Anger in women is almost invariably viewed as 'out of control', neurotic, mad or hysterical. In essence, anger is seen as a mentally unhealthy state.

It is probably the case that the majority of women have difficulties in knowing what to do with their own anger. In consequence, they tend to develop symptoms such as depression, phobias or eating disorders, all of which can be covert expressions of anger (see, for example, Epstein 1987). The racist response to black women who express their anger is to accuse them of having a 'chip on the shoulder', thus implying that their anger is contrived out of an unfounded sense of grievance.

The notion of 'coping' is linked to the tendency among women to cover up and split off unwanted feelings. Hilary Graham (1984) was the first writer to draw attention to the absurdity of this notion and its centrality in women's lives. 'Coping' according to the dictionary means 'contending quietly', implying 'getting things done and not making a fuss'. To be unable to cope, unable to manage day-to-day life without becoming upset, is the thing which many women dread most. Indeed, they have good reason; women who can't 'cope' are likely to lose their children or their liberty.

Poor women and black women in a racist society have a great deal more to 'cope' with than women who are relatively more protected by powerful men. Yet it is precisely those women who are most likely to be censured and punished (for example, by the loss of their children) if they are seen to fail to cope. We have even created a racist stereotype of the black woman as someone who is able to cope with all kinds of hardship and material and emotional deprivation, as though she had no feelings or needs at all. It is against this absurd and hostile stereotype that we tend to measure the actual capabilities of all black women.

The prohibition on the expression of anger and the sense of neediness which so many women feel makes it extremely stressful and difficult for women to tolerate anger and neediness in their own children. While Orbach and Eichenbaum saw in adult women the effects of these difficulties in the mother/daughter relationship, as social workers we are often urged to protect children and disregard the feelings and needs of mothers. In reality, what we are seeing is the real relationship between the situation of women and the care they are able to provide for their children. Most of the cases in which social workers fear that a mother will endanger or neglect her children should be understood as women with an unbearable ocean of unmet needs, all of which are stimulated by the sight of her needy, demanding children.

The effects of material deprivation are clearly crucial in terms of the kind of care a mother will be able to give to her children, both girls and boys. However, I am concerned here to make the point that even a mother who is materially quite privileged is likely to find it difficult to meet the emotional needs of her baby daughter.

The carers and the cared for

Under patriarchy, women are the carers, the nurturers, both for children and for men. In consequence we all learn from our own mothers that we cannot expect very much in terms of care and nurturance for ourselves. It is not that mothers are *consciously* aware of what they pass on to their daughters; on the contrary, many women have every intention of making sure their daughters have a better deal than they have had. But in terms of human relationships, intentions are not enough. Social workers will work with women who desperately want to be good mothers, yet find themselves repeating the pattern of neglect and disregard they experienced from their own mothers. This way of understanding mothering should not be interpreted as women-blaming, however, nor is it a repetition of the cycle of deprivation thesis (Joseph 1972). What it does is to point to the particularly harsh consequences for some women of living in a patriarchal and racist society.

Jean came seeking help at the age of 40. She suffered bouts of depression and had a serious and chronic eating disorder, which had begun ten years earlier, when her daughter was born. At that time, she had had great difficulty in 'mothering' the baby, had wanted to reject her and pretend she had never had a child. The baby's father, with whom she was then living, was perplexed and confused. Social workers and psychiatrists tried to help; Jean was placed in a therapeutic family unit where she gradually became resigned to caring for her baby. However, ten years later, it became clear that nothing had really changed. Jean went through the motions of looking after her daughter, but rarely had any warm or rewarding feelings towards her. Whenever her daughter was at all needy, demanding or upset, Jean became furious. She felt uncontrollably angry and totally bereft.

She felt far too guilty actually to abuse her daughter physically, though clearly her mother's distress was in itself an unbearable pressure upon the little girl. Often Jean would harm herself in some way, express her tears and temper like a tiny child to her daughter's father (with whom she now had only a tenuous relationship) or simply lock herself in her room and cry herself to sleep. Jean's eating disorder, a particularly severe form of anorexia, was her way of punishing herself for what she felt as her monstrous, inhuman disregard of her daughter.

Jean came from a poor, white, country family. Her father was an agricultural worker who worked long hours and left the care of Jean and her younger sister to the sole charge of their mother. The description Jean gave of her mother suggested that she may well have suffered from a mental illness. She was often depressed and preoccupied, subject to uncontrollable violent rages. To Jean, it seemed at times that her mother took delight in hurting and humiliating her.

For Jean, the central paradox of her life was that in spite of knowing how much her mother's behaviour had damaged her, she now found herself doing very much the same sort of thing to her own daughter *and she felt powerless to do it any other way*.

It is interesting to note that Jean worked as a cook and housekeeper. She often worked for very difficult and demanding employers with whom she was endlessly patient and tolerant. Thus, in her working life, Jean continued to be the good daughter, placating her tyrannical mother. It was only in her personal life, and in particular in her relationship with her daughter, that the hurt and furious little girl inside Jean could be experienced.

The attempts to help Jean to 'cope' as a mother, which had proved to be so unsuccessful, were in fact reinforcing the original hurt and deprivation which the little girl had suffered. Instead of addressing the hurt child in her, the workers continually pointed out the needs of her baby and her responsibilities as a mother. Jean was very well aware of these; her problem was that the furious child in her kept preventing her from doing what she knew to be right. What Jean needed was a relationship with a worker in which all the hurt and anger could be re-experienced, taken seriously and to some extent worked through. It was only by working with the hurt child that Jean could be enabled to begin to see her own daughter as a separate person, with legitimate needs which could be met.

Women social workers and women clients

Who is to meet the needs of mothers? Whose job is it to attend to the needy child inside the 'non-coping' woman? While suggesting that social workers are sometimes in a position to do this work, I remain acutely aware that social workers are also very often women. By understanding that women share a common developmental experience, as social workers we have to contend with the fact that we are very much like our clients.

Social workers, belonging to a predominently female profession, are notoriously bad at taking care of themselves, of meeting their own needs. One of the ways in which women learn (as small girls) to set their own needs aside is by dealing with them vicariously, by looking after other people. As women, instead of being fully and painfully in touch with our own unmet needs, we are often inclined to look for people even more needy than ourselves and to make ourselves feel better by taking care of them. For many women, this dynamic provides the unconscious impetus to enter one of the helping professions – nursing, social work, nursery nursing, for example. Most of these jobs offer low pay, bad conditions of employment and little consideration of the emotional stresses involved in the work. This work continues to attract women, not only because at a conscious level it enables women to continue to perform traditional female roles, while getting paid for it, but also because at an unconscious level it is a way in which women deal with their own unmet needs.

Alice Miller makes a useful contribution to this theme in her speculations about what motivates people to become therapists. Miller, who has something of a blind spot around gender, makes no distinction between women and men, but suggests that the person with the greatest natural aptitude for therapy (or social work) will be someone who as a child had to be acutely sensitive to the needs and wishes of her parents. Such children, while their own needs are ignored, develop highly tuned antennae for picking up other people's signals and responding in appropriate ways (Miller 1983). If we reintroduce Eichenbaum and Orbach's contribution here (1983) it seems clear that girls are more likely than boys to become caught up with trying to understand, predict and care for their parents, especially their mothers. This sensitivity to the needs and wishes of others transfers easily into the 'caring' professions. The child described by Alice Miller becomes ever more sensitive to other people, while at the same time becoming more cut off from the feelings within herself of which her parents disapprove (Miller 1981). For a profession such as social work, this is an almost ideal combination!

To generalize, one could say that women who go into social work or other caring professions are very often 'good daughters'; daughters who, from a very early age were good, clean, reliable and helpful, not causing anxiety or distress in their own mothers and in fact repressing the messy, envious, upset, childish parts of themselves.

The roots of child abuse

While a 'caring' job can actually assist with this process of repression, by emphasizing and giving a clear and visible outlet for the adult part of the self, having a child can bring forth quite different responses. For many women, their identification with a baby, especially a baby girl, makes them see in her the split off and never experienced part of themselves. The spontaneity of a baby, and his or her ability to express the full range of emotions, even the 'bad' ones, can make a mother feel full of hostility and hate. While some mothers may actually express their feelings towards their children, many more do not. Instead, they train the child by subtle means, by looks, by disapproval, by shame, until the child learns – as they have done – to be 'good' at the expense of their own feelings. What I am suggesting is that many women, who are on the face of things good carers, do in fact have enormous difficulty in allowing their own children full freedom of expression. A great many women, including some social workers, experience a split between their professional roles, where they are considered as sensitive, tolerant and caring, and what they know of their own feelings towards their children.

Following Alice Miller (1983), I think it is important to consider the point that an inability to tolerate and respond to the emotional needs of children is on a continuum with serious child abuse. While many writers (for example Renvoize 1978) have noted a link between the abusing mother and her own experiences of abuse in childhood, the actual process by which this repetition occurs is rarely articulated or understood by social workers.

Some women, but I suspect a minority, show overt hostility towards their children. Amongst these are the women who, with their children, become the clients of social workers. In working with abusing parents, or even reading the horrifying transcripts of child murder trials, one is often struck by the unrealistic expectations which abusing parents have of their children. We hear of very tiny children being punished for being dirty or untidy, or even for crying. The child is simply being a child; the abusing parent experiences this as hostility, as lack of love. I think this reflects both the often unconscious memories of the parents of the time when far too much was expected of them, but also the thwarted hope that the child will provide the love, care and attention which they lacked. The child is guilty and deserves punishment simply by virtue of being a child and not a parent to its own parents.

Mothers: a case of unconscious child abuse?

I have been speaking here of abusing 'parents', for it is not usually women who abuse children. Yet the question that is often asked when a child is abused by its mother's male partner is: 'Why did she let it happen?' While we know very well that women cannot be held responsible for male violence of which they themselves are victims, we must at least consider the possibility that women do sometimes allow men to hold and express the hostility they unconsciously feel towards their children. Thus the woman can continue to experience herself as the 'good' mother, while unconsciously she allows a repetition on her own children of the abuse she suffered as a child. Some feminist social workers find this idea difficult to accept. We can become so accustomed to defending our women clients by denying they have anything to do with what goes on that we are reluctant to acknowledge the part they may play. Rather than saying, 'The mother didn't know what was going on' or 'How can the mother be expected to stand up to a man?', it might be more useful to look with her at the ways in which she might allow the man, by his abuse, to express the split off and denied part of herself which cannot bear her own children to live in the safety which she did not experience as a child.

This is not to say that women 'collude' in the abuse of their children in the way in which this is usually understood. The notion of 'collusion' is sometimes used to imply that women consciously put the wishes of their partners before the wellbeing of their children. What I am suggesting is that the unconscious, split off part of the woman finds its expression in the physical, emotional or sexual abuse by the man. I do not think I am suggesting anything which makes women rather than men the culprits in child abuse cases. On the contrary, it is my belief that patriarchy, which is strongly supported by male violence, is bad for both women and children. If we are properly to understand how the lives of women and children are affected by the prevailing system, it is important that we do not ignore the dynamic by which women can become involved in perpetuating it.

In thinking about how mothers express and deal with the negative emotions aroused by their children, we have to consider the influence of class and race. It would be wrong to suggest that working-class and black mothers express their hostility through actual violence towards their children, while middle-class, white mothers use the more subtle means which Alice Miller describes. This is simply not true. We know that violence within families crosses class and racial boundaries. However, what we can probably say with some confidence is that we tend to reproduce with our own children the worst aspects of our own relationship with our parents. It is very hard to give to the people you love the most what you haven't had yourself. Much as we might want to do it differently, without help we are unlikely to succeed. It may well be that mothers with a high level of education, who may be in a position to have access to literature on 'correct' child-rearing practices, are less likely to express their hostility overtly.

However, being told that you should not hit your children, that you should allow them freedom of emotional expression, does not change the way mothers actually feel about their children. Indeed, such 'education' may have the effect of making mothers who are already striving to disown their unwanted feelings, push their true feelings even further into repression. If Alice Miller is right, the subtle, shaming, humiliating forms of controlling children are very harmful; they do not just have an effect on the behaviour of children, but actually limit the range of their feelings as well, producing a kind of false self within which nothing authentic can be experienced or expressed.

Sandra: a 'coping' mother

Sandra's story illustrates the way in which a young woman strives successfully to avoid inflicting the worst aspects of her own deprivation on her daughter, but the cost she pays in terms of her own emotional wellbeing is enormous, and in spite of all her efforts her daughter still suffers.

Sandra is a young Afro-Caribbean woman of 22, born in London, who came to the Women's Therapy Centre for help for herself. Her initial complaint was of an eating disorder in which she would regularly overeat and then make herself sick. However, in the course of her consultation with a therapist it became clear that she was often deeply depressed, sometimes suicidal, and that she was rarely able to find anything truly enjoyable in her life.

She is the mother of a two-year-old daughter, and in the eyes of the world she is a most competent person; she is beautiful and charming. She has very little money, but makes a conspicuous effort to dress herself and her daughter well. Sandra's daughter is the centre of her world. Sandra is an excellent manager and a hard worker, though she only ever works hours that enable her daughter to be properly cared for. She has an ongoing relationship with her daughter's father, to whom she remains very attracted. She never knows where she stands with him. She thinks he is very fond of her, and yet he will promise to come around and not come, or arrive late in the evening and then only want to watch television, not talking to her at all. Underneath her competent and charming exterior, Sandra is always on the edge of a terrible depression, sometimes feeling that suicide is the only possible solution. Although she chastises her daughter's father for his behaviour and often threatens to stop seeing him, he knows that really she will always respond to his contrition; in fact as Sandra says, 'he can do as he likes'.

Sandra was the third child of six. Her mother brought the children up alone and was often so overwhelmed by the task that she would go away for days, weeks or even months, leaving the older children to take care of the younger ones. Sandra, according to her own account, was an unattractive child, skinny and plain, with thin hair. Her mother constantly remarked on her daughter's misfortune, and her 'uncle' – by whom she was sexually abused in her early teens – told her that he was only doing this because he felt sorry for her as she was so ugly.

Sandra's little daughter, May, is everything she has always wanted. May is a good girl (like Sandra had been), who is very sensitive to Sandra's unhappiness. She comforts her mother when her father lets her down, even attempting to make coffee and fetch warm clothes for Sandra. In addition, she always tries to please her father when he comes round, in an attempt to get him to take more notice of them.

Sandra's relationship with May's father reflects in many ways the one she had with her own mother. Not surprisingly, she feels totally dependent on someone who really offers her very little. It is as though his very unreliability keeps her stuck there, waiting for him, just as she had to for her own mother. May, although only two years old, is already a 'good daughter'. In fact, she is the ideal mother that Sandra needed and never had. May is constantly concerned for

Sandra and sensitive to her needs. But what has happened to May's own feelings? Already she has learned to cut off from her own spontaneous concerns and focus instead upon her mother's feelings.

Although Sandra has never been offered any help by social workers, her life and her relationship with May, as she herself knows, are far from satisfactory. Mothers like Sandra, who appear to 'cope' so well, who in fact – like little May – learnt to be good mothers from the very start of their lives, are rarely credited with having any needs of their own.

Towards a feminist social work practice

While increasing awareness of women's needs and of issues which are important to women should enable us to plan more relevant strategies, a radical reinterpretation of women's psychology will give us an entirely different attitude to women and to women's needs. There are no easy solutions to offer; the more we understand the kind of deprivation which women suffer and cope with, the more aware we may become of our own and our clients' real and material deprivation.

With an understanding of women's psychology, we will no longer consider coping to be a desirable goal for women, but rather we will be challenging the cost of such coping in terms of women's mental health. We may also ask questions about just why it is that women are being expected to cope. We will often discover that women's coping is the personal, individualized solution to structural social problems, such as poverty, unemployment, the effects of racism and bad health care. This reinterpretation of women's psychology necessitates a re-evaluation of all aspects of social work practice, but it has a specific application to child care practice.

At present, social workers are often asked to implement policies in which the needs of women and children are defined as different and sometimes in conflict. If we can begin to see the continuity of experience of children and women under patriarchy, we will have quite a different understanding of why women sometimes fail to care for or protect their children.

As women working with women, we need to begin by trying to look at our own attitudes to needy women. As 'copers' ourselves, do we unconsciously blame and punish women we see showing that they have difficulties? Nurses very often say that they prefer nursing men to women. This is not because men are easier to care for. It is because women can easily become angry and upset when having to deal with other women who are very needy and vulnerable. All our own split off feelings of wanting to be taken care of can be aroused by our work with women who make great emotional demands on us. We will often find ourselves wanting to minimize the real needs of our women clients, reluctant to hear and engage with the depth of their distress and pain. Often we will have an impulse to collude with the woman's own pretence that she is 'coping', even though we know she isn't.

For the woman social worker, working with very needy, distressed women can present a similar challenge to that of mothering a baby daughter. I think it is quite possible for social workers and other 'caring' professionals to make the mistake of expecting too much of their clients, much as abusing parents often do of their children. Such unconscious abuse of women clients might include, for example, encouraging a severely depressed mother to 'carry on' when our professional judgement ought to tell us that she is simply not able to do so.

In fact, the more we force women to hide and suppress the child in themselves, the less likely they are to be able to offer their children the care they need. Preventive child care should often amount to providing for the emotional needs of women. (Obviously the suggestion is not that we should ignore structural factors, such as poor housing, poverty and lack of day care facilities.) This is precisely what some current child protection policies seek to prevent social workers from offering, stressing instead the importance of identifying 'the high risk family'. The emphasis is often then mistakenly placed on checking and monitoring, rather than doing real preventive work.

One of the biggest obstacles to opening up to the whole area of the emotional needs of women is the sense of shame which our society feels about the needy little children who exist in all of us. To talk to a woman client about the distressed baby inside her, who cannot face the needs of her little daughter, may well be heard as an accusation. To talk to one's senior about the needy little girl inside the social worker . . . well, that, I think, would be a real step forward.

Note

1 See for example, Winnicott, D. W. (1965), *The Maturational Processes and the Facilitating Environment* (London: The Hogarth Press); Guntrip, H. (1986), *Schizoid Phenomena Object Relations and The Self* (London: The Hogarth Press).

References

Baker Miller, J. (ed.) (1973), *Psychoanalysis and Women* (Harmondsworth: Penguin).

Baker Miller, J. (1976), *Toward a New Psychology of Women* (Harmondsworth: Penguin).

Barr, V. (1987), 'Change in women' in S. Ernst and M. Maguire (eds), *Living with the Sphinx* (London: The Women's Press).

Chasseguet-Smirgel, J. (1985), *Female Sexuality* (London: Maresfield).

Eichenbaum, L. and Orbach, S. (1983), *Understanding Women* (Harmondsworth: Penguin).

Epstein, B. (1987), 'Women's anger and compulsive eating' in M. Lawrence (ed.), *Fed Up and Hungry* (London: The Women's Press).

Ernst, S. and Maguire, M. (eds) (1987), *Living with the Sphinx* (London: The Women's Press).

Freud, S. (1964), *New Introductory Lectures on Psycho-Analysis* (Standard Edition 22, 3, London: Hogarth Press).

Graham, H. (1984), *Women, Health and the Family* (Hemel Hempstead: Harvester Wheatsheaf).

Joseph, Sir Keith (1972), Speech to the Pre-School Playgroups Association, 29 June, in E. Butterworth and R. Holman (eds) (1975), *Social Welfare in Modern Britain* (London: Fontana).

Miller, A. (1983), *The Drama of the Gifted Child* (London: Faber).

Mitchell, J. (1975), *Psychoanalysis and Feminism* (Harmondsworth: Penguin).

Olivier, C. (1989), *Jocasta's Children: The Imprint of the Mother* (London: Routledge and Kegan Paul).

Pearson, G., Treseder, J. and Yelloly, M. (1988), *Social Work and the Legacy of Freud* (London: Macmillan).

Renvoize, J. (1978), *Web of Violence* (Harmondsworth: Penguin).

3 *Social work and power relations: towards a framework for an integrated practice*

Marie McNay

Introduction

The past decade has witnessed major economic and political changes in British society. At the same time, there has been a shift to a more personalized emphasis in much social work activity. Social workers have been required to focus on individuals and families 'at risk' and this has led to a more narrow emphasis in defining 'problems'. However, the causes of problems are complex, and related to wider structural processes. Thus it is necessary to reconsider a more integrated understanding of the nature of social problems, and to develop a form of social work practice based on a synthesis of structural and individual (or personal) perspectives. This entails both theoretical work and a more unified approach to the promotion of social work values and principles.

The need to integrate different theoretical perspectives and for an integrated mode of intervention also arises from the wide range of people who become users of social services. Many are, or have been, capable people in many areas of their lives, and their experiences can never adequately be understood by theory. Any theory or idea can provide only a partial explanation of a multitude of complex and interacting factors in people's lives, and one of the most oppressive factors in social work 'practice' has been the way 'theory' has been used. Take, for example, the theory of 'maternal deprivation' which held sway for many years and, despite much criticism, still retains some influence. This theory legitimated the prejudice that a mother's place was at home. By placing the burden of responsibility on the mother, it has been oppressive to women; the status of women who have had to do paid work, especially black and working-class women, has been severely devalued. Thus it is important to challenge such one-sided explanations and find a way either of integrating theories (where they are not in conflict), or transforming them.

This chapter seeks to develop a framework which could facilitate a more integrated mode of intervention based on empowerment. Although the main emphasis is feminist, I am also concerned to understand how feminism intersects with other analyses of inequality, particularly race and class perspectives. There is a need to interrogate theory and to see how various constructions of theory pattern our thinking. Thus, I argue that gender and race perspectives[1] are not just additions to knowledge, but constitute a theoretical breakthrough in understanding the way knowledge is constructed. These perspectives can offer a more integrated understanding of the issues facing social workers, and, rather than negating mainstream theory, suggest possibilities for transforming it. This leads to the development of a broader theoretical framework for understanding inequality and the use of power relations as a unifying concept to understand social relations (while not conflating the effects of different forms of oppression). The framework utilizes systems theory to link the different levels of power as a basis for intervention. Thus, the framework brings together ostensibly disparate strands and offers a new means of forging a link between theory and practice. This mode of intervention does not pose traditional social work methods against alternative or radical methods, but sees the continuities within them (Webb 1981), and utilizes the advantages of both.

Though our particular focus here is on women, the issues discussed in this chapter have wider implications for the theory and practice of social work. My proposal is to work with the wider systems which determine women's lives in order to bring about change which will meet their needs. In the final section, some of the issues are explored utilizing some brief examples from family therapy, to illustrate how the framework could be put into operation.

Issues in the integration of structural and individual perspectives

Approaches to integration

There have been several attempts at integrating structural and individual perspectives in social work education and practice (Evans 1976; Evans and Webb 1977; Corrigan and Leonard 1978; Leonard 1984). These have made important advances, but fall short of developing a framework for a more integrated form of intervention. Pincus and Minahan (1973) and Goldstein (1973) utilized systems theory in attempting to integrate methods of social work. However, this work has, rightly, been criticized for its acceptance of dominant values and consensus assumptions underlying existing social relations (Dominelli and McLeod 1989; Langan 1985; Marchant 1986). Nevertheless, it should be noted that some feminist family therapists have made positive use of systems theory (see, for example, Osborne 1983; Pilalis and Anderton 1986).

Inded, it can be argued that 'systems theory' has no inherent moral or value-laden assumptions, and that it can legitimately be used to describe different social structures. Roger Evans has marshalled an impressive body of evidence to support his view that a consensus model of society is not inherent in the logic of systems theory (Evans 1976: 189). He agrees with Lockwood's arguments (1964) that there has been a failure to distinguish between 'social integration' and 'system integration'. Evans states that the former is concerned with the degree of cooperation or conflict in a society, while the latter is concerned with the causal links of interdependence between groups and institutions. Causal interdependence need not imply social harmony (Evans 1976: 189). Evans supports Mennell's view that the notion of interdependence is 'perhaps the most important contribution of systems theory to social analysis' (Mennell 1974: 190). As we shall see, this notion of interdependence can be harnessed to integrate structural and individual perspectives in social work.

Evans also argued that it was impossible to have an integrated method without an integrated theory. At the time, he argued that an interactionist theory of deviance could be used in exploring the perspectives of 'self' and 'society', and he also advocated the need for a critical social theory. He was not suggesting that it was either possible or desirable to construct an integrated 'grand theory', but rather that it was necessary to adopt a theoretical orientation which saw individuals as dialectically related to social structure, neither wholly free nor wholly constrained (Evans 1976: 193).

Members of the Leicester School of Social Work argued that attempts at establishing integrated approaches had proved premature. In particular, they pointed to the unfulfilled promise of the broad Marxist approach of Corrigan and Leonard, which revealed a 'greater affinity with the social work it was hoping to replace than its authors recognised' (Hardiker and Barker 1981: 268). In the view of the Leicester School: 'Social *theory* for social work was probably impossible in an integrated coherent sense.' They state that what they had attempted was 'to offer the occasional synthesis of a highly segmented activity marked by competing paradigms and epistemological discontinuities but, more properly viewed, the exercise stands in terms of social *theories*' (Hardiker and Barker 1981: 268). They made an important contribution to social work by explicating theories for use in practice, but they remained 'atheistic' about a social work metatheory. However, they retained some allegiance to the possibilities of synthesis (Hardiker and Barker 1981: 269).

Feminism – the construction of theory and social work practice

The most significant work in integrating the structural and the individual levels of analysis, the personal and the political, or the private and the public, has been carried out by feminists. In view of this it is surprising that feminism has had such an apparently marginal effect on social work theory and practice, when it has so much potential to contribute to an understanding of social relations (Hudson 1985). However, Sue Wise (1985) comments on the 'silences' of feminist analysis in helping her work with the everyday problems of a social services department. I believe that these contrasting statements lead to two key issues in understanding why feminism has had such a marginal impact on social work. First, theory used in social work is constructed through a sexist process, and second, feminist social work practice is largely perceived as being work with women.

The first issue, the sexist construction of theory, has been increasingly exposed by feminist analysis of the gendered assumptions which underpin much theory formulated in a male-dominated society. This process has parallels with the ethnocentric nature of most theory formulated in a white-dominated society (though I am not suggesting the processes have the same effects). By looking at 'theory' from feminist/gender and race perspectives, the ways in which thinking is structured by dominant values become clearer.

Feminist theory, like theories about 'race' and 'racism', are (if they are addressed at all) usually 'added in' as areas of study in various educational courses. Critiques of some 'main' teaching areas may be provided by adding pieces of work by feminist and black authors, but these often appear to pose simply 'another' view. It is rarely recognized that both gender and race perspectives offer fundamentally different outlooks on social relations. Both types of analysis have developed important theoretical tools which question conventional views of social relations. They also provide concepts and categories for transforming existing theories. For example, the book *Good Enough Parenting* contains the following statement:

> The group were asked to consider the needs of children up to early adolescence, a period in which the assertion of independence and the struggle to separate from families is a major preoccupation (CCETSW 1978: 11).

This statement incorporates a conventional theory of adolescence (the term itself being a construct). However, the period during which children grow into adulthood may be different for girls and boys and different for girls and boys from different races and cultures. 'Separation' may take a different form for girls and boys, and in some cultures, it may not happen at all. A gender perspective would focus on the way in which boys are usually encouraged to make their way in the world as breadwinners, while girls may be encouraged to help in the home, thereby having less 'separation' from the parental figures (especially mother). In some cultures, children never leave the parents' household (particularly in the case of female children) or simply move from one household to another, acquiring a new set of parents by marriage. Some children grow up in several households and have several parent figures. Thus, the concept of independence, or growing autonomy, must be considered in a culturally specific and gendered way. In using gender and race/culture perspectives, the categories for analysis, e.g. 'independence', 'separation', are transformed, demonstrating how the theoretical tools of gender and race can contribute to the revision of mainstream theory.

Although the author of the statement (CCETSW 1978) quoted earlier acknowledges the need to challenge cultural assumptions (but not gendered assumptions), he is nevertheless unaware of how deeply embedded in our everyday lives certain constructs are. The experience of living in a white- and male-dominated society means that not only are social structures pervaded by certain norms and values, but our whole process of thinking is structured by the prevalent ideas of society. The structure and the process interact and reinforce each other. Most theory formulated in white Western society attempts to explain social phenomena within an overall framework of norms and values which have held sway for centuries.

Gender and race perspectives question an exploitative sexual division of labour and oppressive relations between white people and black people, i.e. existing power relations. Looking at 'our' social structure and processes from this viewpoint, it is easy to understand why feminist and radical social work practice are marginalized. Those who put forward such perspectives are accused of lacking the 'objectivity' of conventional wisdom and of seeking to 'indoctrinate' people. It is difficult for people who have lived all their lives believing in the current social system and its broad norms and values to understand that they themselves have been subject to indoctrination. In this respect, the current trend towards anti-racist social work is a challenge to traditional theory and practice. It is not surprising that such initiatives are often perceived in liberal equal opportunity terms rather than as any threat to the status quo. What 'equal opportunity' means is open to a variety of interpretations and the term is also generalized across a range of areas – age, gender, sexual preference, class, disability, race, culture and creed (CCETSW 1989: 3).

Gender and race analyses are not just another addition to ideas but, together with a class analysis, they can provide a theoretical framework for transforming our understanding of social relations. In the field of social work, their theoretical tools can help us understand inequality, structured by social divisions of gender, race and class, and the social problems which emerge within unequal power relations. While other forms of discrimination need to be addressed, they are not central to the structured inequality essential for the profit base of our current economic relations, as are the divisions of gender, race and class. There are diversities and commonalities in the experience of people subject to unequal power relations (Hanmer and Statham 1988). However, the theoretical tools for understanding power relations in general can provide an overall framework within which particular forms of oppression can be analysed. In this way, structural and individual perspectives can be integrated, since power is manifested at all levels of people's lives. Using such a framework does not mean throwing out all the 'theory' currently used in social work. What it does mean is that present theory can be transformed within a clearer, more unified understanding of particular goals and values. The revision of mainstream theory is crucial not only to the demarginalization of feminist social work practice, but also to the whole process of developing 'good' practice in social work, that is, empowering all people who experience oppression.

The second issue in relation to marginalization is that although feminist analysis is concerned with the oppressed position of women, it does not follow that feminist practice is concerned only with women. Feminist family therapy is one area, for example, where work is being tackled with women and with the significant people in their lives. More similar practice developments are necessary if feminist practice is to be demarginalized. Wise has pointed to the difficulties of working with different groups of vulnerable people where, for example, helping an oppressed mother might be at the expense of a vulnerable child (Wise 1985). Yet such needs may not be contradictory. Whereas traditional social work would usually focus on tackling the problem of the mother's 'parenting skills', a feminist approach would begin from a different definition of the 'problem', particularly the wider issues in unsatisfactory relations. This may mean encouraging the woman to develop her own potential, while sharing child care. The more satisfaction she can achieve for herself, the more likely it is that she will be able to provide 'good' parenting.

This example illustrates that it is often not easy to distinguish 'feminist' social work practice from good practice generally. (See Hale 1983; The Birmingham Women and Social Work Group [81] 1985; which deploy a variety of ideas, not all of which are feminist). Feminist analysis is insufficient on its own, but practice which does not counter women's oppression (i.e. use the insights of feminism) cannot be good practice. The same is true of anti-racist social work; good social work must be anti-racist.

'Feminism' can, and should, encourage change that enhances all members in relationships, though this is not always possible. Feminist practice developments need to tackle the complexity of the inter-relationships of the various vulnerable and oppressed groups. Feminist practitioners must show how their insights can be used by other workers who do not yet understand the relevance of feminist analysis for the range of problems with which they have to deal.

A unified value system

In order to develop an integrated practice, it is necessary to have a unified value system. Principles and values in social work have always given rise to heated debate. Some principles, such as confidentiality, are regarded as ideals not easily attained, while values conflict according to theoretical and political positions. For example, one of the main principles of social work, that of self-determination, has been consistently criticized as unrealistic in a society based on inequality and social divisions which limit most people in achieving their potential. This principle was redefined as 'self-realisation' in the British Association of Social Work (BASW) Code of Ethics (adopted 1975 and revised 1976), as Joan Baraclough argues, in order to recognize the limitations which real-life situations impose (Baraclough 1976). Hence, it is necessary to address these issues in the process of developing an integrated social work practice. We need a more unified approach to the promotion of social work values and principles. It is now generally acknowledged that principles of equal opportunity are central to social work and these principles should form the basis of a more unified value system.

Formulations concerning the values of social work, set out in the 1989 CCETSW document on the Diploma in Social Work, propose that social workers should have 'a commitment to social justice and social welfare, to enhancing the quality of life of individuals, families, and groups within communities, and to a repudiation of all forms of negative discrimination' (CCETSW 1989: 10). To achieve professional qualifications, social workers are required to 'recognise the need for, and seek to promote, policies and practices which are non-discriminatory and anti-oppressive' (CCETSW 1989: 10).

The document marks a major shift in conceptualizing the nature of social work and social problems by acknowledging the processes of structural oppression in society, particularly in relation to race, class and gender (CCETSW 1989: 10). Many leading figures in the formal organizations of social work have embraced equal opportunity principles, particularly in response to the pressure of anti-racist activities. What we need now is to develop mechanisms that can help us translate the new values into action. The unifying concept of power offers the possibility of developing a framework of intervention consistent with the values of social justice. The acceptance of the idea that unequal power relations are the basis of social injustice provides the foundation to use the concept of power, to develop a broad organizing framework within which more specific understandings can be formulated. This will help us review existing 'theory', to develop a more integrated approach to the promotion of social justice and a better social work practice.

The tendency in more critical approaches to mainstream theory and practice (for example, in some forms of radical social work) has been to 'throw the baby out with the bathwater'. This has tended to encourage false polarities. However, a framework which utilizes the concept of power can span the various dimensions of structural power and personal power and the inequalities and differences within different social relations. Thus, structure, culture and biography can be analysed in a more integrated process.

Power relations: a framework for analysis

There are two key elements in the framework: power relations and systems theory.

The concept of power relations

Sophie Loewenstein argues that: 'Power has replaced the Freudian libido as the overall integrating motivational concept for all human behaviour' (Loewenstein 1976: 92). She states that: 'The relationship between men and women, between races, between different social classes, and between helping professionals and their clients are all variations of unequal power relations in society' (Loewenstein 1976: 92). She is aware that these relations differ for each group, but that there are also some common denominators. She suggests that power relations provide a unifying concept of human behaviour in modern society and she shows how traditional theories can be re-examined in the light of power relations to develop a more integrated understanding of human behaviour. Though Loewenstein focuses on an

American college curriculum, and the method is different from that suggested here, the main themes are still useful in moving to a different organizational framework for social work teaching and practice in Britain.

I would formulate a definition of the concept of 'power relations' as follows:

> Where relations are so structured that one person or group of people benefits at the expense of another person or group of people, then the people who benefit can be said to have greater power in those relations. The power can be manifest at an individual, family, group, community or societal level and can take material and emotional forms.

Power may be exerted in a wide range of forms: material, emotional or ideological. Using power relations as a unifying concept necessitates an exploration of the dimensions of power whenever we consider explanations of social issues. It may not be necessary or appropriate to reject particular theories, but rather to understand how being set in a wider context of power would change their meaning. Thus, for example, in considering theories of 'mothering', the quality of care given may be understood in terms of the personality of the mother or in terms of her powerless social situation or through the interaction between both factors. Exploring this interaction will result in a more integrated understanding. It will then be possible to consider more specific theories about oppression. For example, in relation to race, if the mother was black, then it would be necessary to examine how racism might impact on her capacity to provide care. (See Barbara Solomons 1976, for a very useful portrayal of the relationship between power, powerlessness and the processes of human growth and development in relation to black people.) The impact could have positive or negative effects, promoting strong links of family solidarity against adversity or resulting in conflict and difficult relations.

The framework of power relations exposes values which underpin much mainstream social work theory and practice. It offers critical insights into processes of social interaction which may be taken for granted, and reveals assumptions which are often implicit in traditional social work practice. For example, Western orthodox theory of the family often assumes middle-class, nuclear family norms. The work of Salvador Minuchin, exemplified in a basic text (Minuchin 1974), illustrates this type of theorizing. In his approach to family therapy, Minuchin invests authority in the father figure rather than the mother, and in parents rather than grandparents. Taking a power relations approach makes explicit his assumptions about gender roles, since it highlights how power is invested in the man and how he ignores a wide range of cultural patterns to do with the extended family, where grandparents are often the major authority figures. This example is not unusual, since family structures reflect wider structural processes in society; hence the relevance of systems theory.

Systems theory and power relations

Power is manifested at different levels and connected within different structures of society. Systems theory can link these different levels through the notion of the interdependence of systems. In systems theory, any combination of interacting elements can be understood as an organism comprised of different parts, or sub-systems, which are interdependent in the overall functioning of the whole. Applied to societies by the functionalist school of sociology, systems theory explains how any society must have some degree of coordination and integration among its constituent elements or social institutions, and attempts to demonstrate how the central value system of society is reinforced through the institutions.

This analysis has been applied to the family as a social institution. Parsons and Bales (1956) demonstrated how the process of socialization operates within the family system to pattern the personality of the child to the needs of the wider social system. The dependency of the young child makes it particularly subject to the influence of the values of parents who are themselves integrated into the cultural value system of society. Parsons and Bales use Freudian theory to show how, in American society, the social differentiation of the sex roles is established, the man taking the more instrumental role (in external affairs) and the woman taking the more expressive role (in internal affairs). Hence they view the family as a powerful unit of social control. This type of analysis has been elaborated further by other functionalists. Bell and Vogel (1960), for example, describe the interchanges between the family and personality systems and other social systems, namely the economy, the polity (government), the community and the societal value system.

Systems theory can be applied to any society, regardless of its particular norms or values, since it *describes* an interaction process. It is particular theories which provide the *analysis* of the society and which are underpinned by particular values and a theoretical perspective which may explain social interaction in terms of consensus or conflict. Applying systems theory to social work reveals how values in the wider society interact with social institutions like the family and social work agencies. Systems theory also clarifies the ways in which the distribution of power in macro social-structures is reflected and reinforced in micro social-structures like the family. Thus, for example, the sexual division of labour in the economy, where men predominantly have status and power, is reflected in the sexual division of labour in the family, where men often hold power, particularly in major areas of decision making (Gillespie 1972). Though the inter-relations between these processes are complex, material and ideological power have a major bearing on emotional power, and it is this interaction that needs to be understood.

Therefore, a systems approach can help to develop a more interactional framework, while the power relations approach, particularly utilizing analyses from gender, race and class perspectives, shows how theories can be transformed to develop a more integrated analysis of social issues. Thus, this framework can be utilized to develop an approach based on different values and different analyses than the ones with which most mainstream practitioners might currently work, yet still utilize mainstream theories and techniques. Since a power relations perspective assumes conflict in social relations based on inequality, then this framework proposes a mode of intervention to work with power, conflict and change, the overall objective of which is to transform power relations.

A mode of intervention based on empowerment

Social work has tended towards a problem-oriented mode of intervention. This can be a useful way to work with specific issues, but it raises problems of 'problem-oriented' theorizing. One problem is the relative lack of theories to explain how people who are thought to be managing their lives reasonably successfully actually do it, and how other people develop considerable coping skills in the face of all sorts of adversities.

Another problem is the tendency not to see people as whole people who need to get satisfaction in their lives. Thus, a narrow focus on an issue like parenting skills can ignore the wider issue of the emotional investment good parenting requires and that such investment is hard to give if people have little good experience to draw on themselves. This tendency can also be detected in work with people classified as mentally ill, mentally handicapped, elderly, and so on. They are often seen as 'schizophrenic', 'geriatric', and so on, rather than *people* who have particular problems.

A further argument for a different mode of intervention arises from the wide range of people who become clients. Since most social work theory is drawn from analysis of dysfunction, situations can be over-theorized and straightforward approaches overlooked. Many users' situations do not require complex theorizing, and in those which do, this could be undertaken at a later process of intervention rather than at the outset.

The proposed mode of intervention is based on the recognition that everyone has basic needs (though these are mediated differently in different cultures) and that if these needs are not met, then certain functions will be harder to carry out. Hence, it is not users' 'problems' which need to be assessed but what resources (emotional or material) and skills are required to meet their needs. The assessment may begin from more simple concepts but may require more complex theorizing as obstacles to realizing needs become clearer. This mode of intervention is about a way of approaching situations, about certain values in promoting social justice and about seeing people as people. It is geared to the process of realizing needs and to the development of techniques and strategies to facilitate this. The definition of 'need' itself is complex, but this approach is premised on developing mutual perceptions/understanding between user(s) and worker(s). Any use of theory would come from the mutuality of dialogue between both parties, so that 'theory' is constructed from people's experience.

Many social theorists have emphasized the need to see theory and practice as inter-related processes, with the dialogue between user(s)/interviewee(s) and worker(s) as central. This has become one of the tenets of radical social work (for example, Leonard 1975) and a basic tenet of feminist research practice (for example, Stanley and Wise 1983). Social workers need a great deal of 'theory' and knowledge to engage with users in making 'sense' of their situations. However, there is a dilemma here for workers. If their analysis is inaccurate, too narrow or premature, it may be unhelpful or even damaging. If there is no analysis, then users may not get the help they need. Thus workers have to construct the analysis from people's experience, holding ideas and knowledge as prompts until shared understanding develops between user(s) and worker(s). This process of constructing, testing against practice and reconstructing theory has been called praxis. Dialogue and praxis are essential to a non-oppressive mode of working, and it is vital to recognize that our understanding is always tentative and partial.

This mode of working draws on the power relations framework to help people articulate their needs and to understand what blocks them from realizing such needs. It is geared to developing the positive aspects of people's situations rather than focusing on the negative aspects, and to helping people gain more control, and thereby more satisfaction, in their lives. It utilizes a range of theories for analysing situations, transformed by the power perspective and linked to different levels and structures of society. Thus, it is based on empowerment, since it entails helping people work with their power relations and with the interdependent systems within which they operate.

Intervention: power, conflict and change

Social structures continually change, and social workers are always working with dynamic situations. The systemic perspective has been utilized in family therapy and this, together with some of the techniques employed, provides useful ideas in working with change. In the remaining part of this section, I will explore some issues related to change. I will then develop two aspects of intervention – building self-esteem and confidence and working with resistance and change – to indicate the kind of development that is possible within this mode of intervention. The theoretical issues already outlined provide the analysis for the situations, and the techniques offer ways of intervening to bring about change.

i) SYSTEMS AND CHANGE

A key notion within systems theory is the idea that systems are either 'open' or 'closed'. Open systems are concerned with growth, hence tension and conflict are endemic to them. Closed systems operate in such a way as to reduce strain in the system. These concepts are used in family therapy to suggest that 'open' systems go on developing to meet new contingencies in life, while 'closed' systems are resistant to change. The degree to which a family system is open or closed depends on the inter-relationships of the individual personality systems within the family system, and the family system within wider social systems. However, as no social system can remain static, understanding the dynamics of systems can be useful in assessing both factors, i.e. increasing resistance as well as opening up potential for change. Because even systems which are thought to be at the 'closed' end of the continuum will experience tension if they are resistant to change which is inevitable, these ideas are useful in considering how tension and conflict can be utilized to promote different relations.

Traditional forms of intervention in social work are premised on the assumption that a consensus exists between the needs of individuals and families and the society within which they live. A power relations perspective exposes the unequal and inherently conflictual character of social relations. Thus, we need to develop a different approach to working with conflict to create different social relations rather than the ones which preserve the status quo. My approach is to work with change that can enhance all members in relationships. This includes tackling the resistance of the more powerful to their loss of power but works with the potential of gains for all.

ii) BUILDING SELF-ESTEEM AND CONFIDENCE

Helping people to develop self-esteem and gain more confidence to control their lives may require a variety of resources, including training, but the initial steps often have to be taken in personal relations.

The starting point is the acknowledgement that people have basic needs, for example self-esteem, praise, recognition, and achievement, and if these needs are not met, then their capacity to control their lives will be diminished. Thus, the assessment aims to identify what people want and how they propose to achieve the goals identified. This approach focuses on what skills and resources people have, or have tried to use, to achieve their needs, rather than how problems have developed which can reinforce the powerless position. Thus, for example, in some relationships, including family relationships, it may be a simple form of communication that is required. People often do not express what they want or communicate positive feelings, and some situations can be resolved by using communication techniques. The emphasis here is on the development of skills to get more satisfaction from social relations in a variety of contexts. It recognises that there are both positive and negative forces in people – mixed feelings (or ambivalence). The object is to reinforce positive aspects of relations, in the hope that the negative aspects will recede or be perceived differently. Even if the negative aspects do not diminish, it is essential for people to feel they themselves have some value, or can feel they have some good things potentially, in order to tackle the more negative aspects of their lives.

The work of David Wilmot (1977) aims to help people to feel good about themselves. He attempts to bring out the positives in situations, helping people express what they want, rather than what they don't want, which is more usual. He uses a variety of techniques, including games and exercises, to help people communicate their needs and aspirations.

This type of approach can be productive, since many people 'compete' in family and household relationships (just as individuals compete in the capitalist economy). Such competition can increase stress and minimize further the capacity of people, particularly 'mothers', to meet others' needs. Facilitating communication, strengthening the capacity to make decisions and helping people resolve conflicts are ways of working with change. Exposing unmet needs, particularly with women, can produce other kinds of conflict but, simultaneously, produce ways forward that signal hope and alternative ways of living lives. All members of households are responsible for the quality of their relations and the running of the household. Therefore, members have to learn to cooperate over tasks, share resources, and learn that they are more likely to get satisfaction if they do not compete and achieve at someone else's expense. Cooperation over tasks is particularly important for single parent households, though linking into wider systems and support networks is also crucial.

Work in building the confidence of people in themselves and with each other should also expose the source of conflicts. Many conflicts internal to household systems are caused by the external systems, for example low income. Clarifying such issues can help people relocate the conflict and direct their energy where the source of the problem exists, i.e. not to take it out on each other but to work on the social institution which is responsible.

iii) WORKING WITH RESISTANCE AND CHANGE

Freud's concept of defence mechanisms as a defence against anxiety is an important tool for social workers in tackling resistance to change. It can be utilized to understand the source of some conflicts and how anxiety and resistance can be reduced. However, the degree of resistance to change in any person depends on her or his power within a system. In this context, some other techniques of family therapy may be useful.

Systems theory shows how difficult it is for one member of a system to change if other parts of the system do not also change. For example, Longres and Bailey (1979) argue that men's concerns need to be understood as well as women's if sexism is to be eliminated. They note that family counselling has been used to renegotiate marital contracts in the direction of greater equality, but they acknowledge that sexism is rooted in male privilege and that change will not come about without a struggle. It is the way struggle is conducted which can open up the potential for change.

The effects of power differentials on decision-making in marriage (Gillespie 1972) and how satisfaction in marriage is viewed differently by women and men (Bernard 1976) can be made explicit with techniques from systemic family therapy. The technique of circular questioning (Palazzoli *et al.* 1980), where the views of one person are sought concerning the relationship between two others can be used to bring out different perceptions or world views. Or, asking one person to express how s/he thinks another person thinks or feels and then checking the accuracy of the opinions can also reveal important differences or conflict. These techniques, used after confidence-building techniques, if necessary, can help people hear information they may not have heard before which can help them to perceive situations differently. However, it is essential that alternative ways of conducting relationships are built into the work, so that people are able to see their way out of the conflict. The people who have most to lose need to be clear what it is they are able to gain (for example, a happier partner who will be able to meet other needs) if they are to give up some of their privileges.

The 'restructuring' techniques used by Minuchin and his colleagues (1974; 1981) are useful to help people practise change within the interview situation, as well as at home, and to get people to experiment with different patterns of relating. Ideas that might be resisted in the abstract are often adopted when tried out in practice, because the ideas can be seen to work and have benefits. A particular technique – 'unbalancing' – is used to change the hierarchical relationships between members (though within dominant norms already noted), by 'unbalancing' the system. This technique is aimed at empowering a family member low in the hierarchy by creating an alliance to challenge his (*sic*) prescribed position in the system. This can then produce changes which develop new realities and consequently, 'a change in the perspective of family members in relation to what is permissible in the transactions among members' (Minuchin and Fishman 1981: 162).

Perhaps the most useful conceptualization of change and its processes has been formulated by Watzlawick *et al.* (1974). They pose two different types of change: first-order and second-order change. In first-order change, change occurs within a given system which itself remains unchanged; in second-order change the system itself changes, i.e. requires changes in the body of rules governing the structure or internal order of the system. Watzlawick *et al.* show how attempted solutions (first-order change) can maintain the problems. They use second-order change techniques to move the situation out of what they consider is a contradictory position or trap, i.e. to reframe the attempted solution. They also suggest that their principles for change can be applied at many different levels of social systems. This formulation is often applied to what appears to be small aspects of change on the basis that change can be effected most easily if the goal of change is reasonably small. The experience of change then leads to further change. This approach is very useful in countering behaviours which maintain problems and current relations, and offers techniques for changing the rules of the way the system operates, and hence the power relations.

I have considered working with resistance as it may block change but, clearly, there are many forms of resistance which bring about change. Space limits the development of such strategies here but they can be seen as 'the other side of the coin' – both forms of resistance complementary and intertwined in the processes of change.

Family therapy techniques can help people change in relation to their immediate system by utilizing the dynamics of change within the system itself. However, some people are unable to use some of these types of intervention, and what blocks them from using such opportunities needs to be understood and other forms of intervention offered. Some people may need to bring out deep-seated conflicts before they are able to move on in their social relations. The approach offered here still provides the broad organizing framework within which to examine power relations in these situations, but more complex theorizing about emotional development may have to be utilized.

Conclusion

The aims of this chapter have been work towards a framework which could help social workers organize their thinking in order to integrate various conceptual levels, explore ostensibly competing theories and develop an empowering mode of intervention. The ideas are tentative and need further work, but I hope there has been sufficient exploration and illustration to help workers to rethink some of the traditional approaches.

The approach has a central concern for women, but suggests that women can often be helped by a focus on the power relations and systems within which they are structured. The contention is that these social relations need to change if women are to achieve and maintain satisfaction in their lives.

Note

1 'Gender' and 'race' are complex terms and require some clarification. I use the term 'gender' perspective to refer to analyses which explain female/male relations as they are socially constructed; this includes feminist analysis. The term 'race' perspective is more problematic, because it is historically connected to the development of racism. However, I use it to embrace ideas and concepts of ethnicity and culture usually rendered invisible in mainstream texts. I use the term 'race' rather than 'ethnicity' to acknowledge that the effects of racism are central to any discussion of these issues. I also use the term 'culture' to signify that a variety of 'cultures' exist among ethnic groups, that it cuts across concepts of race and class, and that 'culture' is not a static notion.

References

Baraclough, J. (1976), *A Code of Ethics for Social Work* (London: BASW).
Bell, N. W. and Vogel, E. F. (1960), 'Towards a framework for functional analysis of family behaviour', in Bell and Vogel (eds), *A Modern Introduction to the Family* (London: Routledge and Kegan Paul).
Bernard, J. (1976), *The Future of Marriage* (New Haven: Yale University Press).
Birmingham Women and Social Work Group (81) (1985), 'Women and social work in Birmingham', in E. Brook and A. Davis (eds), *Women, The Family and Social Work* (London: Tavistock).
Brook, E. and Davis, A. (1985), *Women, The Family and Social Work* (London: Tavistock).

CCETSW Study 1 (1978), *Good Enough Parenting* (London: CCETSW).
CCETSW Paper 30 (1989), *Requirements and Regulations for the Diploma in Social Work* (London: CCETSW).
Corrigan, P. and Leonard, P. (1978), *Social Work Practice Under Capitalism: A Marxist Approach* (London: Macmillan).

Dominelli, L. and McLeod, E. (1989), *Feminist Social Work* (London: Macmillan).

Evans, R. J. (1976), 'Some implications of an integrated model of social work for theory and practice', *British Journal of Social Work*, 6, 2.
Evans, R. J. and Webb, D. (1977), 'Sociology and social work practice: explanation or method?' in *Contemporary Social Work Education* 1, 2, August 1977.

Gillespie, D. L. (1972), 'Who has the power? the marital struggle', in H. P. Dreitzel (ed.), *Family, Marriage and the Struggle of the Sexes* (New York: Macmillan).
Goldstein, H. (1973), *Social Work Practice: A Unitary Approach* (University of South Carolina Press).

Hale, J. (1983), 'Feminism and social work practice', in B. Jordan and N. Parton (eds), *The Political Dimensions of Social Work* (Oxford: Blackwell).
Hanmer, J. and Statham, D. (1988), *Women and Social Work: Towards a Woman-Centred Practice* (London: Macmillan).
Hardiker, P. and Barker, M. (1981), *Theories of Practice in Social Work* (London: Academic Press).
Hudson, A. (1985), 'Feminism and social work: resistance or dialogue', *British Journal of Social Work*, 15.

Langan, M. (1985), 'The unitary approach: a feminist critique', in E. Brook and A. Davis, 1985.
Leonard, P. (1975), 'Towards a paradigm for radical practice', in R. Bailey and M. Brake (eds), *Radical Social Work* (London: Arnold).
Leonard, P. (1984), *Personality and Ideology* (London: Macmillan).

Lockwood, D. (1984), 'Social integration and system integration' in G. K. Zollschon and W. Hursch (eds), *Explorations in Social Change* (London: Routledge and Kegan Paul.

Loewenstein, S. F. (1976), 'Integrating content on feminism and racism into the social work curriculum', in *Journal of Education for Social Work* 12, 1.

Longres, J. F. and Bailey, R. H. (1979), 'Men's issues and sexism: a journal review', in *Social Work* (USA) 24, 1.

Marchant, H. (1986), 'Gender, systems thinking and radical social work', in H. Marchant and B. Wearing (eds), *Gender Reclaimed* (Sydney: Hale and Iremonger).

Mennell, S. (1974), *Sociological Theory, Uses and Utilities* (London: Nelson).

Minuchin, S. (1974), *Families and Family Therapy* (London: Tavistock Press).

Minuchin, S. and Fishman, H. C. (1981), *Family Therapy Techniques* (Harvard: Harvard University Press).

Osborne, K. (1983), 'Women in families: feminist therapy and family systems', in *Journal of Family Therapy* 5, pp. 1–10.

Palazzoli, M. S. *et al.* (1980), 'Hypothesizing, circularity, neutrality: three guidelines for the conductor of the session', in *Family Process* 19, 1.

Parsons, T. and Bales, R. F. (1956), *Family, Socialization and Interaction Process* (London: Routledge and Kegan Paul).

Pilalis, J. and Anderton, J. (1986), 'Feminism and family therapy – a possible meeting point', in *Journal of Family Therapy* 8, pp. 99–114.

Pincus, A. and Minahan, A. (1973), *Social Work Practice: Model and Method* (Illinois: F. E. Peacock).

Solomons, B. B. (1976), *Black Empowerment: Social Work in Oppressed Communities* (New York: Columbia University Press).

Stanley, L. and Wise, S. (1983), *Breaking Out: Feminist Consciousness and Feminist Research* (London: Routledge and Kegan Paul).

Watzlawick, P., Weakland, J. and Fisch, R. (1974), *Change: Principles of Problem Formation and Problem Resolution* (New York: W. W. Norton).

Webb, D. (1981), 'Themes and continuities in radical and traditional social work', in *British Journal of Social Work* 11, pp. 143–58.

Wilmot, D. (1977), 'Problem families – problem therapy', handout from a training session, self-published.

Wise, S. (1985), *Becoming a Feminist Social Worker*, Studies in Sexual Politics 6 (Manchester: Department of Sociology, University of Manchester).

4 *Who cares? Women in the mixed economy of care*

Mary Langan

Introduction

Financial constraints, political pressures and the attentions of the mass media have, over the past decade, transformed the climate in which the personal social services operate. The results have affected the lives of the women who make up the large majority of both staff and clients of local authority social services departments. At a time of wider economic insecurity and a shift in public opinion to the right, the restructuring of social services has had a differential impact, not only on women members of staff and clients as compared to men, but also among women themselves, according to their social class, ethnic and sexual identity and whether they are disabled.

Two themes have proved particularly influential in guiding the transformation of the personal social services. The first is the promotion of the family as a key agency of care and control in society. While attempting to sustain the traditional nuclear family, public policy has been increasingly directed towards regulating the more diverse family forms that have resulted from the demographic and social changes of recent decades. The enforcement of a specifically gendered division of labour in the new family forms, as well as the assumption of ethnocentric family norms, remains central to official family policy.

The second theme is the restructuring of local authority social services departments according to the principles of the new 'mixed economy of welfare'. The objective is that the local state should no longer be regarded as a *provider* of services, but as an *enabler*, promoting the provision of packages of care by combinations of private firms, voluntary organizations and informal care in the home, in association with a residual public sector. The reorganization of social services according to commercial principles is likely to polarize staff between a thin layer of social work experts, managers and accountants on the one hand, and a mass of deskilled care workers on the other. It is also likely to cut back public provision for many of those most in need – poor women and their children, older women, minority ethnic groups, people with disabilities, and special needs groups such as people with HIV/Aids. Before examining the operation of these themes in the specific policy areas of child care and community care, let us look at each in more detail.

The regulation of the family

Government policy on the family presents an apparent paradox. On the one hand the restructuring of public provision in the spheres of income maintenance, housing and health as well as social services has withdrawn support from the family (Alcock and Lee 1988). Public welfare services have been undermined at a time when wider economic trends encouraged by the government – notably persistent unemployment and demographic changes, particularly the growing proportion of older people – have imposed greater demands on family life (Henwood 1990; Langan 1990). On the other hand Conservative governments have made support for the family and the promotion of traditional family values central ideological themes (Langan 1988).

To resolve this paradox it is important to grasp the subtlety of new right pro-family rhetoric. Though this involves considerable emphasis on sustaining or reviving the values of the traditional nuclear family, it also includes an acknowledgement of, and an accommodation to, the reality of more diverse extended family forms. What is taking place is an extension of the traditional nuclear family paradigm to incorporate a new model family. Critics who focus one-sidedly on the traditionalist emphasis of Tory rhetoric underestimate the elements of discontinuity concealed by the appearance of continuity; elements of the old model are preserved while others are superseded. This process deserves closer scrutiny.

The model family of modern capitalist society assumes a close conjugal relationship between a male breadwinner, and a female homemaker who carries the major responsibility for rearing their two or three children (Elliott 1986). The nuclear family norm is sustained by legislation (notably in relation to divorce), by official taxation and social security policies, and by the whole structure of welfare provision (Land 1978; Smart 1987). The personal social services and the profession of social work emerged in the post-war period to support those few 'problem families' which could not (or would not) maintain the nuclear norm (Clarke, Langan and Lee 1980).

The nuclear family model has long been a focus of feminist critique because of its oppressive consequences for women. It endorses women's dependence on men, their exclusion from the public world of work and their confinement to the private world of housework and child care (Langan 1985). Feminists have also increasingly exposed the divergence between the nuclear model and the reality of growing single parenthood, family breakdown and diversity (Coote, Harman and Hewitt 1990). Anti-racist critics have challenged the way the nuclear model assumes not only the universality of the white Anglo-Saxon family form, but also assumes its normality and superiority. As a result the more diverse extended family forms of the Irish, Afro-Caribbean and Asian communities have been labelled as deviant, and devalued (Ahmed, Cheetham and Small 1986; Dominelli 1988). The oppressive consequences of the ideology of the nuclear family have been a recurrent theme of lesbian and gay discourse over the past twenty years (Weeks 1985).

In recent years, however, the nuclear family has not only been criticized by radicals, it has also been undermined by changing social trends. According to a major survey compiled by the Family Policy Studies Centre 'the nuclear family is undergoing extensive change' (Kiernan and Wicks 1990: 18). The authors summarize the most significant changes as fewer marriages, more cohabitation and extra-marital births; increases in divorce and remarriage; declining fertility and smaller families; and the rise of one-parent and reconstituted families. They conclude that 'although the nuclear family is still the most prominent form, the nuclear family is for increasing numbers of individuals only one of several possible family types that they experience during their lives' (Kiernan and Wicks 1990: 18).

Another factor weakening the traditional nuclear model is the growth in female participation in the labour market. Whereas in the 1930s only 10 per cent of married women went out to work, fifty years later 60 per cent had jobs (Kiernan and Wicks 1990: 26). This contrast is less striking for black women, who have always tended to have a higher rate of participation in the labour market than white women. Whereas black women tend to work full-time, many of the newly created jobs taken up by white women were part-time (Barrett and McIntosh 1985). Numerous surveys have confirmed that the complementary emergence of the 'new man' who takes his fair share in domestic and child care tasks remains a fiction. Where women work full-time, they still do the bulk of caring for children and older relatives (Henwood, Rimmer and Wicks 1989; Wicks 1990).

There are two aspects to the official response to the decline of the nuclear family. The first is to bolster up the traditional model through propaganda and policy measures. The second is to recognize changing realities and to modify policy to take account of the new diversity of family structures. As we shall see, the former outlook in the end predominates in the government's approach to child protection, where the emphasis is on traditionalist ideology; the latter takes priority in the sphere of community care for older people, where major demographic changes generate demands for resources which necessitate a more pragmatic and practical policy.

'Around 1977 both main British political parties began to place the idea of "supporting the family" at the centre of the political agenda, and it is not difficult to detect the economic pressures which lie behind this' (Finch 1989: 125). The advance of pro-family ideology can be traced from the first major drive to reduce public expenditure on welfare in the post-war period under James Callaghan's Labour government in the late 1970s. Conditions of economic austerity prompted the revival of traditional family values of sharing and caring. In the Thatcher years, official statements repeatedly emphasized traditional family ideology in relation to a wide range of social policy issues. Such statements and the resulting public discussion about issues of child-rearing and parenting present parental relations in apparently neutral terms. Yet they conceal highly gendered assumptions about appropriate paternal and maternal roles.

The 1990 White Paper on crime emphasizes the disciplinary responsibilities of parents in relation to their children:

> Crime prevention begins in the home . . . From their children's earliest years parents can, and should, help them develop as responsible, law-abiding citizens. They should ensure that their children are aware of the existence of rules and laws and the need for them; and that they respect other people and their property. Most parents try to carry out these duties conscientiously. When effective family control is lacking, children are more likely to grow up without self-discipline and a sense of concern for others. They are more likely to commit crimes (Home Office 1990: 40).

After this homily on traditional family values, the White Paper adopts a more menacing tone: 'When young people offend, the law has a part to play in reminding parents of their responsibilities.' Another way in which the government has promoted the doctrine of parental responsibility is in the use of income maintenance regulations to enforce the dependence of 16- and 17-year-olds on their families (Family Policy Studies Centre 1988).

A further illustration of the government's drive to sustain traditional family norms is the pursuit of errant fathers, which Margaret Thatcher made a personal crusade:

> Government, too, must be concerned to see parents accept responsibility for their children. For, even though marriages may break down, parenthood is for life. Legislation cannot make irresponsible parents responsible, but it can and must ensure that absent parents pay maintenance for their children *Margaret Thatcher 'The Pankhurst Lecture' given to the '300 Group', 17 July 1990 (*The Guardian *18 July 1990).*

Mrs Thatcher proposed the establishment of a 'child support agency' to hunt down the guilty men and compel them to pay up. The October 1990 White Paper *Children come first* revealed the government's plans to make fathers pay up to half their disposable income in child support payments (Department of Health 1990).

The former prime minister's focus on not merely *parental*, but specifically *paternal*, responsibilities reflects a more general concern of government policy to restore the traditional authority of the *father* in the nuclear family. In recent years patriarchy has come under threat not only from the growth of single parenthood and divorce, but also from advances in reproductive technology (Smart 1989; Birke *et al.* 1990). In vitro fertilization has created the possibility of separating reproduction not only from marriage but also from paternal control. Traditional parenthood has come under threat from lesbian and surrogate mothers conceiving by artificial insemination with donor sperm. Furthermore, traditional fatherhood, always assumed to follow from the legal contract of marriage, can now be confirmed – or challenged – by the new technique of genetic fingerprinting.

The state has tried to bolster up paternal rights. The 1989 Children Act promotes paternal rights by encouraging unmarried fathers to claim parental rights and responsibilities. This undermines the scope of autonomous motherhood and potentially puts sperm donors in the same position as unmarried fathers. At the same time a married mother who has artificial insemination from a donor is allowed to register her husband as the baby's father, while no such protection is extended to an unmarried mother. Thus unmarried women who have artificial insemination are at risk that their anonymous sperm donor might claim paternal rights (Smart 1989). Government proposals to allow children born as a result of AID to trace their biological fathers, and to allow biological parents continuing access to their children whom they have given up for adoption, are further indications of official anxiety at the erosion of the significance of biological paternity (*Sunday Times* 23 September 1990).

The final and most significant area in which public attention has been focused on parental/paternal powers and responsibilities is that of child abuse, or more specifically, child sexual abuse. A national debate about child sexual abuse erupted in 1987 in response to events in Cleveland. Here a sudden dramatic increase in diagnoses of child sexual abuse by a newly appointed paediatrician working in cooperation with a specialist social work team resulted in a large number of children being removed from their families. A major local campaign asserted parental and, above all, paternal rights against state interference in 'normal' family life (Bell 1988; Campbell 1988). In presenting the subsequent official report by Lord Justice Butler-Sloss to parliament, Tim Devlin, the junior minister responsible referred to the 'current unpleasant situation in which an over-zealous local authority that suspends disbelief finds it easier in law to take away a man's (*sic*) children than to suspend his bank account' (*Hansard* 6 July 1988).

The common theme in all these instances is the authorities' concern to sustain the traditional nuclear family model in face of forces that threaten to undermine it. However, another aspect of government policy comes to the fore if we shift our attention from the sphere of children, born and unborn, to that of older people and others, such as people with mental illness and learning difficulties, and people with disabilities, who are often placed in a state of dependence on the care of others. Here we discover that a different model of the family has come to play a growing influence, though often implicit and understated, in the formulation of government policy. The family model that underpins much of the 'community care' policy of the 1970s and 1980s is that of the 'modified extended family', defined as 'a coalition of nuclear families in a state of partial dependence' (quoted in Finch 1989: 124).

The sustained drive to reduce institutional care for people with mental illness and learning difficulties as well as the repeatedly proclaimed commitment to caring for older people and others in need 'in the community' all assume the existence of extended kinship or neighbourhood networks that can provide the necessary support (Langan 1990). Income maintenance and social services policies are designed to put pressure on 'liable relatives' or household sharers to take on some of the burden of care. For example, meals on wheels or home helps are much less likely to be provided for an old person who lives with a relative or shares the same roof with another person (Parker 1990). The extended family or neighbours are expected to help with cooking, shopping and other domestic tasks (Abrams *et al.* 1989).

The introduction of the Invalid Care Allowance in 1975, the only financial support available for caring, was widely criticized because, until a judgement by the European Court against the British government in 1986, this benefit could not be paid to married women, who constituted the great majority of eligible carers. Yet the very provision of this grant to carers other than the conventional dutiful daughter reflected the shift of official policy towards an implicit endorsement of more diverse family forms.

While the nuclear family model has long been the target of feminist and anti-racist critique, the problems of the new model are only beginning to be appraised. Janet Finch has argued that the 'modified extended family' should more accurately be labelled the 'gendered modified extended family' to draw attention to the oppressive consequences for women of their enhanced role in informal (unpaid) care in the community (Finch 1989: 125). Finch notes the curious alignment of traditional right-wing support for self-help in the family and neighbourhood, and the radical critique of institutional care, which emphasizes decentralization, client autonomy and deprofessionalization. She insists on the importance of making visible the unpaid labour of female carers.

From the perspective of minority ethnic families, the new recognition of the legitimacy of extended family forms may appear progressive. But in the context of the withdrawal of resources for supporting families, such recognition is likely to prove merely another justification for forcing black and minority ethnic families to continue 'looking after their own' as they have always been obliged to do (Rooney 1987).

Both aspects of state policy towards the regulation of family life have had important implications for social services departments and the practice of social work, to which we now turn.

The restructuring of the personal social services

A number of commentators have argued that the term 'mixed economy of welfare' implies a false counterposition between the (private) sphere of the capitalist economy which operates according to rigorous free market principles and the (public) world of welfare which caters simply to social need (Walker 1984; McCarthy 1989; Knapp 1989). Ever since the emergence of the welfare state in the 1940s, the profitable expansion of private capital has always set an external limit on public expenditure on welfare. For the same period, welfare benefits and services have been provided through a mix of private and public mechanisms. Walker writes of a continuum in which the two extremes rarely appear in a pure form, and of 'vague and shifting' borderlines in a complex 'social division of welfare' (Walker 1984: 19–26). Knapp distinguishes four sectors of supply (public, voluntary, informal and private) and six varieties of demand, producing a '24-celled matrix' offering 'a bewildering variety' of ways of delivering and financing welfare (Knapp 1989:

23). What is less well-recognized is that all sectors of the mixed economy of welfare rely heavily on the labour of women, whether paid in diverse caring occupations, or more commonly, unpaid in the home (Pascall 1986).

Two key factors have changed the framework of the welfare state and shifted the boundaries between public and private, formal and informal. Firstly, ever since the end of the long post-war expansion in the recession of the mid-1970s, successive governments have squeezed public expenditure in an attempt to reduce the burden on private profitability. The decline of British capitalism has constrained the provision of welfare across the board. Secondly, since Mrs Thatcher's first general election victory in 1979, the government has proclaimed a strong ideological commitment to rolling back the state sector, opening up nationalized industries and welfare services alike to the wider operation of private market forces, and to an even greater contribution from the voluntary and informal sectors.

For a time the personal social services were protected from the full impact of government austerity measures by local authorities which cut housing and education first. However, the combined effect of the continuing financial squeeze and measures to curtail the autonomy of local government resulted in a steady decline in the rate of growth throughout the 1980s. The practice of imposing cash limits led to underspending and undermined planning and innovation (Baldock 1989; NALGO 1989). This sluggish growth in resources must be set against the steady increase in demand resulting from demographic and economic trends and from the increasing scale of child abuse, family breakdown, domestic and racial violence, drug abuse and HIV/Aids infection.

The first indication of a major government offensive on the personal social services came in a speech by health minister Norman Fowler in Buxton in 1984. In this speech Fowler first outlined the government's project of fostering an 'enabling role' for social services departments in planning, monitoring, supervising, regulating and supporting a range of private, voluntary and informal welfare services, rather than playing a major role as service providers. He also emphasized the need to use existing resources more efficiently and recommended attempts to attract resources from businesses, charities and voluntary groups. He proposed the more extensive use of charges (for services such as home helps and day centres) and the privatization of particular services (McCarthy 1989).

The message of Buxton was amplified in the Audit Commission's 1986 survey of community care, which, although highly critical of the government's poorly-planned closure of long-stay institutions, echoed Fowler's demand for greater 'value for money' in social services departments. In 1988 the Griffiths report on community care outlined a comprehensive programme based on the application of the spirit of Buxton to local authority social services departments. What are the consequences of these developments for social work?

By the close of the 1980s the personal social services and the mainstream social work profession were in a state of shock:

> It is hard now to remember the sense of optimism, the belief in the capacity of social workers to make a real impact on the lives of the vulnerable, disadvantaged and disturbed, that characterised the time between the publication of the Seebohm Report (1968) and the advent of the social services departments (1971) (Bamford 1990: ix).

The emergence of the 'generic' social worker as the key figure in the newly created local authority social services departments was one by-product of the liberal social reforms of the 1960s. Twenty years later the world of social work had become more sceptical in its outlook and more pessimistic about the scope for progressive social change.

Conflict and demoralization were already becoming widespread in social work in the late 1970s, when the tensions between growing demand and stagnating resources became more and more apparent (Clarke, Langan and Lee 1980; Smith nd). Public debate polarized between right wingers who blamed social workers for subverting individual responsibility and social cohesion, and radicals who accused them of facilitating the reproduction of oppressive capitalist social relations. While social services managers took advantage of the cuts to reimpose discipline and to restrict the scope of services, radical social workers looked to community groups, women's organizations, anti-racist movements and diverse self-help organizations to pursue their transformative ideals. The emergence of a feminist perspective on social work, followed in the 1980s by the development of the anti-racist movement in social work, marked the beginning of the new era of anti-discriminatory practice (Wilson 1977; Dominelli 1988; Langan and Lee 1989).

By the early 1980s the ideological attack on social work had become increasingly virulent (Brewer and Lait 1980; Anderson 1980). Right-wing social policy commentators denounced social workers as hopelessly ineffective, and demanded their abolition or radical reorganization. When the proposals of Thatcher's Family Policy Group were leaked in 1983, it appeared that the cabinet itself endorsed these views. Prominent social policy academics, such as LSE professor Robert Pinker, adopted a notably defensive posture, making major concessions to the new right critique (Pinker 1985). In the climate of austerity and vituperation that surrounded social work in the early 1980s, the Barclay Committee attempted to bridge the gap between Seebohm's radicalism and the rampant reaction of the 1980s, and inevitably failed. Its compromise concept of the 'community social worker' was rejected by Pinker, in a minority of one on the committee (Barclay 1982).

Though Pinker was dismissed as an 'emasculated social democrat' and more recently as 'a lone voice', as the 1980s proceeded his approach converged with that of the government (Leonard 1982: 79; Baldock 1989: 47). Pinker now proposes that social workers reduce their horizons to 'task-centred, problem-solving, crisis intervention, and behaviour modification methods' (Pinker, nd). Despite the unpopularity of many of his views within social work, it is likely that Pinker anticipates the trends of the 1990s. Government pressures to curb local authorities, and its determination to extend market forces, as well as the general reaction against the legacy of the 1960s, all point in a similar direction. If social work does have a role in the 1990s it is, at least in the eyes of the government and influential policy experts, as a more specialized service, with a more restricted vision of its role in promoting empowerment and equality, but with a more active role in regulating family life and promoting the mixed economy of welfare. There is little place in this perspective for developing the feminist or anti-racist dimensions of social work practice.

The restructuring of the personal social services by the more rigorous application of market principles is likely to reinforce the existing hierarchical sexual and racial division of labour. Though women constitute only 63 per cent of all local authority workers, they account for 87 per cent of social services staff (Hallett 1989). Howe's survey of the state of affairs in the late 1970s drew attention to the tendency for women to be concentrated at the lower levels of the social services hierarchy, while men dominated senior positions. In 1977 some 83 per cent of social work assistants and 64 per cent of social workers were women; at every other level from team leader/senior (49 per cent women), through area officer (29 per cent women), divisional area officer (17 per cent), men predominated (Howe 1986).

More recent figures show that little has changed. Still, more than 90 per cent of directors are male and more than 70 per cent of area officers are men (Popplestone 1980; Foster 1987). The LACSAB/ADSS 1988 survey shows an increasing feminization at the lower levels of the social services hierarchy: 74 per cent of social workers and 90 per cent of social work assistants are women. This marks the culmination of a trend already noted in the early years after Seebohm, when the 'young Turks' influenced by the radical social work movement began to replace the 'old Maids' associated with traditional casework (Davis and Brook 1985). This trend has been reinforced by the (male) managerialism of the 1980s (see Lupton in this volume). Paradoxically, the growing feminization of welfare has been accompanied by the further masculinization of the social services hierarchy.

At the very lowest level of the social services hierarchy – care and domestic staff in homes and day centres, home helps, and other domiciliary care workers – women make up around 75 per cent of staff (Howe 1986; Jones 1989). In many areas, manual employment in social services departments provides poorly paid work for white women. In other areas, especially in the inner cities, significant numbers of black women are employed in these jobs (Jones 1989).

Black people appear to be under-represented at every level of the social services hierarchy. Though no national statistics are available on the ethnic composition of the social services workforce, local surveys suggest that relatively few black workers are taken on, especially at higher levels (Rooney 1982; 1987; Hughes and Bhaduri 1987). Statistics on minority ethnic entrants into relevant training courses confirm continuing racial bias. Though there has been some increase of black recruitment on to social work courses: 'For candidates holding similar qualifications, applicants from the majority ethnic group are more likely to be successful in taking up a place on a course than those from minority ethnic groups' (CCETSW 1985: 17). There is still a marked under-representation of minority ethnic students on post-qualification specialist courses (CCETSW 1986–89).

Changes in training and qualifications for social services staff may consolidate the existing gendered and racialized hierarchy. In addition to the new Diploma in Social Work, an 'advanced award' in social work can now be conferred upon 'advanced' practitioners and social services managers. This award is intended to ratify trends towards more specialist social workers, particularly in the fields of child protection and mental health, where post-qualification courses and dedicated teams are already widespread. The advanced award is intended to encourage the emergence of staff trained in the managerial and commercial skills necessary in the new-style 'enabling' social services department. Meanwhile, for social care staff, a new Certificate in Social Care is planned.

Attempts to raise professional standards and to provide better vocational training for manual staff are undoubtedly to be welcomed. One of the virtues of the new proposals is the way that they begin to recognize care as a skill, rather than as a taken-for-granted female attribute. However, it is important to point out the danger that they may simply reinforce the prevailing polarization between an overwhelmingly white male management and a predominantly female staff. It is striking for example that although many women social workers have moved into the child protection speciality, their advance has been paralleled by that of their male colleagues into the managerial hierarchy where they retain power and authority. Though social work authorities have proclaimed a commitment to providing improved access to minority ethnic applicants, this may not counteract the structural discrimination that tends to prevail in the existing system.

Child care

The 1989 Children Act provides a useful, if complex, illustration of the direction of government social policy in a sphere of great importance for social workers and for women in general. It attempts to create a new framework for child care and protection at a time when issues such as child abuse, family breakdown and single parenthood have become the focus of heated public controversy. A number of commentators have noted the contradictory character of the legislation as an instrument of social policy (Frost and Stein 1990; Parton 1991). Here we discuss the consequences of the Children Act for women in the light of the approach to child care and protection which seems likely to come to the fore. The Act attempts to reconcile demands from prominent inquiries into cases of physical abuse (London Borough of Brent 1985; London Borough of Greenwich 1987; London Borough of Lambeth 1987) for a more interventionist and coercive approach from the public authorities and those of the 'parental rights' lobby which mobilized so effectively in response to Cleveland. The Act also reveals the application of the government's enthusiasm for the market to the sphere of child welfare. The Act reflects both the state's attempts to regulate family life and its desire to reduce the public contribution to child care.

By contrast with earlier legislation, the Children Act acknowledges new family forms and relationships, including unmarried parents and step-relationships. It repeatedly urges local authorities to give due consideration to a child's religious persuasion, racial origin and cultural and linguistic background (Department of Health 1989). However, despite all the sensitive wording, the traditional conjugal couple and their parental relationships, in the end, predominate. When the Act repeatedly refers to the family as the best place for the child, it is clear that the ethnocentric nuclear ideal is assumed. Even where the conjugal relationship has ended and the couple are living apart, the Act emphasizes their continuing *parental* relationship to the child or children. This emphasis on parental responsibility as something shared between mother and father reveals underlying assumptions and evasions about motherhood, fatherhood and the white nuclear family which have important consequences for women and their children.

The Children Act assumes that motherhood is a natural and ennobling state, ignoring the whole issue of women's subordinate position in family life. It neglects the often oppressive reality of women's role as houseworker and mother in the absence of adequate social support facilities. The Act upholds the virtues of paternity, yet evades all the associated problems of male power, male sexuality and the socialization of masculinity. Yet these are the forces that maintain men's power over women and children within the family, and are central to the prevalence of child sexual abuse. Focusing on the pathological family or the deviant father distracts attention from the oppressive patriarchal relations of the 'normal' family, the problematic character of conventional male sexuality and its close links to domestic violence (Feminist Review 1988). The Act assumes that the privatized world of the conjugal family, within which women take the major responsibility for intimate relationships and child care, is the ideal arrangement within which to rear children. It gives no rights or recognition to lesbian parents, independent or joint mothering, or indeed any 'deviant' parenting arrangements.

In its broader approach to child care policy, the Children Act embodies a dual strategy. On the one hand, it emphasizes the responsibility of the statutory authorities to identify children *in danger* and take the appropriate measures to protect them. The new legislation shifts power away from local authorities and social workers in favour of the courts. At the same time it places specific responsibilities on social services departments to adopt a more active investigatory role in relation to families at risk and to work in close collaboration with other agencies, including the police. On the other hand, the Act establishes a framework for providing supportive and preventive child care services for children *in need*. This involves a voluntary partnership between the family and the state in which the family acts as a consumer of a range of services, such as accommodation, day care and social work support. These services are to be provided either directly by the state, or by other agencies coordinated by the local authority social services department. The government has moved away from any concept of providing universal welfare services as a right to all children in accordance with market forces.

In developing the legalistic aspect of official policy towards child protection, the influence of the NSPCC, and in particular of the work of its innovative Child Protection Team at Rochdale, Lancashire has been considerable (Dale *et al.* 1986; Parton and Parton

1989). In sympathy with the ascendant right-wing drift in social work, Dale and his co-workers explicitly reject the traditional liberal and supportive approach to abusing families followed by the NSPCC, as indulgent and likely to encourage dependency. They propose a much more robust 'modern' approach, emphasizing control and authority. They are sharply critical of the hesitancy of much social work with families at risk, an approach they characterize as 'professional dangerousness', which risks compounding the problems of abusing families. Adopting an American model of 'therapeutic control', the Rochdale team follow a method of 'intensive engagement', carefully but rapidly distinguishing truly 'dangerous families' (from which children should be permanently removed) from not-so-dangerous families (which should be encouraged to carry on without social services interference).

The Children Act envisages the expansion of the private, voluntary and informal sectors in providing for the special needs of children who are physically and mentally disabled or socially disadvantaged. It welcomes the development of such a mixed economy of welfare in the provision of accommodation, day care and services such as family centres, holiday and travel schemes. The government is keen to clarify two distinctions here. The first is that between children who need day care or accommodation as a welfare service and those whom the courts decide require council care as a protective or coercive measure. The Children Act abolishes the former catch-all category of 'voluntary care', which often obscured this distinction. The second distinction is that between the welfare needs of targeted children in need and those of children in general. Thus, while local authorities retain responsibility for children with special needs, children who require day care simply because their parents are working are being pushed into the care of private nurseries and childminders or obliging grandmothers. Hence as the private and voluntary sectors expand, the children who remain reliant on local authority services will be those from the poorest families often with the greatest needs. While private provision flourishes the most disadvantaged children will be 'selectively' accommodated in a residual, stigmatized, and under-resourced public sector.

Former health minister Edwina Currie summed up the government's commitment to promoting private enterprise in child care and reserving the public sector for targeted children with special needs:

> Our view is that it is for the parents who go out to work to decide how best to care for their children. If they want or need help in this task, they should make the appropriate arrangements to meet the

> costs. Our objective is that there should be a range of day care services so that parents can make a choice. Public provision by local authorities should concentrate on the particular needs of children from families with health or social difficulties (*Hansard* 12 July 1988).

The deregulation of day care for the over-8s and the introduction of charges for the under-8s indicates the direction of government policy (Redding 1989).

In the climate created by the Cleveland cases, the sponsors of the Children Act held back from fully endorsing the interventionist and coercive approach recommended by the Rochdale team. Indeed it is striking that the Act, with its emphasis on the welfare of the child, its focus on parental responsibilities (rather than parental rights), and its concern to establish independent complaint and appeal procedures, retains many progressive features. As we have seen, it also encourages the expansion of preventive and supportive services for families. However, the Act's conception of prevention is narrow, based on targeting particular families in need, rather than providing universal child care facilities that would reduce the strains of child care on families in general and mothers in particular. It is also worth noting that the supportive aspects of the Children Act are permissive, whereas its coercive features are obligatory. As funding for local authority social services declines, social workers will be obliged to carry out the statutory aspects of the Act, such as maintaining registers of children at risk and appropriate levels of surveillance, while general support services are neglected.

It is striking that these pressures were already evident as the Children Bill made its way through parliament. As Parton has observed, the effect of introducing a child assessment order *as well as* an emergency protection order (at first only the latter was planned) is that 'rather than reducing the likelihood of increased state intervention in the family, it may have increased' (Parton 1991: 243). Despite the progressive image of the Children Act, as time passes the hard face of the Rochdale NSPCC may very well come to the fore. The impact of both the more authoritarian drift of child protection policy and of growing austerity in the provision of public services are likely to fall most heavily on mothers, particularly if they are working class, single or black.

Though the Children Act comments neutrally on 'parenting', in reality it is mothers in inner city areas who will become the main target of tighter control and surveillance (C. Parton 1990). The adoption of technical/bureaucratic methods, including abuse registers, specialist teams and inter-agency collaboration, means in practice closer supervision of poor families (Frost and Stein 1989).

The widespread use of Greenland's checklist method of identifying 'high-risk' families illustrates the dangers of the intrusive approach to child protection in the absence of wide-ranging resources for prevention and support. In 1987 Greenland extended his earlier attempts to identify 'dangerousness' among mentally ill and violent offenders to 'lethal family situations' (Greenland 1987; Parton and Parton 1989: 62). He lists nine factors for both parents and child which correlate with a high risk of abuse; if a family scores above 50 per cent for either parents or child, the risk is designated as high.

Greenland's criteria of high risk are strongly biased against working-class and black families. On the grounds of poverty, poor housing, early marriage and child-bearing, many working-class parents would be well on the way to qualifying as high-risk. Add single parenthood and many Afro-Caribbean families would automatically come under official surveillance (Channer and N. Parton 1990). Greenland's checklist takes no account of the wider material conditions and power relations which lead to abuse, or indeed of the resilience of working-class family structures which enable them to withstand the difficulties of bringing up children in straitened circumstances. This is even more the case in relation to black families, where both the pressures of racism and the strengths of black parenting are underestimated.

The fact that the highly publicized Beckford and Henry cases involved black families provoked a wave of racist commentary in the media. Social work intervention in these families revealed the influence of equally dangerous stereotypes. The notion that the Afro-Caribbean extended family can cope with all the problems of child care without external support was one such assumption. The myth of the all-coping black mother helps to legitimize the failure to provide adequate child care services. On the other hand there is the danger of cultural relativism. A social worker may believe that beating young children is the norm in some minority ethnic communities and fail to take appropriate action to protect a child (Channer and N. Parton 1990). Another difficulty is to recognize the barriers to the disclosure of physical or sexual abuse in communities for which the family provides a vital source of support and resistance against a racist society. In such cases disclosure of abuse means opening the family up to direct intervention by racist state authorities (see Hudson in this volume). It is not surprising that some of the sharpest conflicts between black communities and social services are about issues of child care and parenting. As a result black children are over-represented in various forms of state care and the prejudice that the black family is pathological has become firmly established in British society, not least among many social workers (Roys 1988; Bryan in this volume).

Working-class and minority ethnic women are also likely to be the main victims of the residualization of local authority services. Women living in poor areas, often dependent on income support and living in high-rise flats or poorly resourced estates, will suffer most from reduced council services. They will benefit least from the expanding private and voluntary sector, which will flourish in middle-class areas and cost more than many women can afford. They will inevitably be forced to carry a greater share of child care in the home. In cases where women physically abuse or neglect their children, high prevalences of poverty, depression, isolation and fatigue have been recognized (C. Parton 1990). An increased incidence of abuse and neglect as a result of more intensified deprivation seems almost inevitable.

The Children Act proclaims a partnership between the state and families to promote the best interests of children. The question of how far it is possible for the state to act in this constructive way on behalf of women and children has aroused considerable controversy within feminist and radical opinion in social work and beyond. Linda Gordon (1986) rejects the traditional dogmatic anti-state position, arguing that state intervention can shift power inside families, towards women and children and away from their male abusers. Carol Smart (1989), however, takes the view that such alliances can be a mixed blessing for women as the resolution of the conflict rarely takes place on women's terms. Most feminists recognize that, whatever their reservations about the police, the courts and social workers, there will always be situations in which the protection of women and children from male violence must justify state action. In cases of sexual abuse, feminists in practice emphasize official support for the mother and child against the abusing male.

Can the Children Act be used judiciously by feminist social workers to help women and children? There are strong grounds for doubt. The Children Act reveals little understanding of, or sympathy for, the feminist perspective on power relations and child abuse. Indeed its sympathies seem to lie rather with protecting paternal authority. The events at Cleveland and elsewhere have revealed a widespread and deeply rooted reluctance to accept the high prevalence of sexual abuse in families. Despite all the evidence, to accept the scale on which male relatives sexually abuse children involves too great a threat to the paterfamilias. Given the lack of recognition of family power dynamics in the Children Act, it is by no means clear that it will prove useful in tackling the real problems of abuse. However, the Act does include provisions to assist the perpetrator of abuse to move out of the family home. Though this provision is rather ill-defined it marks a significant shift from the conventional practice of removing – and implicitly blaming – the child victim.

Community care

Whereas the significance of the Children Act lies largely in its ideological focus on traditional family values, the NHS and Community Care Bill, introduced into parliament in January 1990, acknowledges changing family forms and seeks to take advantage of extended kinship networks. Furthermore, while the child care legislation has limited consequences for the restructuring of personal social services, the full implementation of the government's community care plans will fundamentally change local authority social services departments and the practice of social work. Though the government announced in July 1989 a two-year delay in funding these proposals in order to keep the newly introduced poll tax down, local authorities have in general pressed ahead with their community care plans.

Under the new community care legislation the local authority social services department will no longer be a 'monopolistic provider' of services. Instead it is to become an 'enabling authority', assessing needs, designing community care 'packages', securing service delivery and monitoring quality. The new entrepreneurial social services department is supposed to promote 'cost effectiveness' and to encourage competition among providers, giving preference where possible to the voluntary and private sectors. The logic of the government's community care plans is to privatize much of local authority social services, reducing the role of the social services department to that of managing the remainder. The end product will be a two-tier welfare system in which the private and voluntary sectors look after anybody who can raise the required funds, while the local authority deals with a residuum of the poorest and the most difficult. The result is likely to be a decline in the accountability of 'arm's length' service providers and an under-resourced directly managed service (Langan 1990).

Anti-racist and feminist voluntary groups which seek to involve and empower client groups and to challenge prevailing welfare norms have responded apprehensively to the new legislation. They are concerned that they will no longer be able to act as innovators, to speak as advocates of the interests of service users, or to campaign against the authorities. The replacement of grants with long-term contracts which stipulate conditions in a more detailed and formal manner gives greater power to the local authorities and curbs independence and local initiative. For these groups the crucial feature of the new legislation is that, at a time when the demand for all forms of social care is on the increase, it proposes changes in the administration and funding of community care without recommending any increase in overall resources available (Hall 1989; Thompson 1989).

Anti-racist organizations have criticized the bill for failing to make the provision of community care more responsive to the particular needs of black and minority ethnic communities. Ratna Dutt has called for positive action to encourage the provision of contracts to black and minority ethnic groups:

> Until packages incorporate the black and/or anti-racist dimension, then black communities will continue to be marginalised and 'care' will continue to be the sham it is now (Dutt 1989).

The National Council for Voluntary Organizations (NCVO) has emphasized the need for wider information and consultation, and has set up a Community Care Project with a particular concern to ensure that the concerns of black and minority ethnic groups are taken into account (NCVO 1989).

Despite the long-asserted demands of feminists and other campaigners for more support for carers, the government's community care plans offer only familiar platitudes about creating opportunities and offering respite care. The Act makes no specific recommendations in the sphere of income maintenance or in relation to encouraging access to wider involvement in the life of society. Recent changes in income maintenance and welfare policy are likely to make matters worse rather than enhance carers' capacities for an independent life (Langan 1988). The community care Act virtually ignores the now widely acknowledged fact that the vast majority of carers are women, and fails to take account of demands for alternatives which do not exploit women. The government has remained deaf to Janet Finch's argument that 'women must have the right not to care, and dependent people must have the right not to rely on their relatives' (Finch 1988: 30).

Pioneering schemes in Kent and Gateshead, which anticipate the policy shifts encouraged more widely by the government's community care plans, illustrate the consequences for women in the family and in social services departments (Challis and Davies 1986; Ungerson 1990). These schemes seek to mobilize maximal support for the 'frail elderly' in the community, often taking advantage of existing family or neighbourhood networks. These networks are supplemented by the efforts of 'community care helpers', who enjoy no employment rights but are paid a token amount according to tasks carried out rather than by hours spent. Such schemes assume the continuing subordination of women, not only in the family, but in the wider community mobilized to support older people at home. In the Kent scheme 94 per cent of the helpers were women and pay was maintained below tax and income maintenance thresholds. At the same time this approach encourages the proliferation of a deskilled, predominantly female, social services workforce as market forces march ahead into the sphere of community care.

Conclusion

After more than a decade of austerity and reaction, any survey of contemporary trends in social work and social policy and their impact on women inevitably reveals a rather bleak picture. Yet it also reveals contradictions in official policy and important points of contestation. In both the main areas we have examined – child protection and community care – elements of a renewed feminist agenda and a new approach to anti-discriminatory social work practice are beginning to emerge.

Christine Parton has surveyed the feminist approach to child protection work in both voluntary and statutory agencies, emphasizing the themes of prevention, protection and, where appropriate, rehabilitation. To prevent child abuse, particularly sexual abuse, it is necessary to challenge male sexuality and the socialization of masculinity in all areas of social life. This should include, for example, sex education in schools, an area neglected by the Children Act. In the sphere of protection, removing the father should take priority over removing the child, while resources should be made available for intensive therapeutic work with mother and child. The emphasis here should be on empowering women and enabling them to break out of their dependent and vulnerable position (Parton 1990; see also Hudson in this volume).

In a similar way, Janet Finch has indicated the main elements of a feminist agenda in community care. The first priority here is pushing demands for more support for female carers. Measures which make it easier for both female and male workers to carry out their caring responsibilities, and forms of community care which encourage more men to take on unpaid caring tasks should also be promoted. Feminists also need to challenge the assumptions about the family that underlie the community care consensus, arguing that 'community care need not mean family care'. The provision of care in a range of residential and day care facilities, by properly qualified and well paid professionals, is essential to relieve the pressures of community care on women, both in the home and in the social services department (Finch 1990). This approach must go hand in hand with a real commitment to user self-determination – we should not forget that the majority of cared-for people are also women.

In all spheres of welfare an anti-racist dimension must become inseparable from promoting a feminist perspective in social work practice. The narrow outlook of radical social work in the 1970s, which neglected both gender and race issues, contributed to the ascendancy of the new right in the 1980s. If we are to regain the initiative in the 1990s, the broader vision of anti-discriminatory social work is vital for all women in all spheres of welfare.

Acknowledgement

I would like to thank Fiona Williams and John Clarke for their comments on a draft of this article.

References

Abrams, P., Abrams, S., Humphrey, R. and Snaith R. (1989), *Neighbourhood Care and Social Policy* (London: HMSO).

Ahmed, S., Cheetham, J. and Small, J. (1986), *Social Work with Black Children and their Families* (London: Batsford).

Alcock, P. and Lee, P. (eds) (1988), *Into the Third Term: Thatcherism and the Future of Welfare* Social and Urban Policy Papers 1 (Sheffield: Sheffield City Polytechnic).

Allen, N. (1990), *Making Sense of the Children Act 1989* (London: Longman).

Anderson, D. C. (ed.) (1980), *The Ignorance of Social Intervention* (London: Croom Helm).

Audit Commission (1986), *Making a Reality of Community Care* (London: HMSO).

Baldock, J. (1989), 'United Kingdom – a perpetual crisis of marginality', in B. Munday (ed.), *The Crisis in Welfare: an International Perspective on Social Services and Social Work* (Hemel Hempstead: Harvester Wheatsheaf) pp. 23–50.

Ball, C. (1990), '*The Children Act 1989: origin, aims and current concerns*', in P. Carter, T. Jeffs and M. Smith (eds), *Social Work and Social Welfare Yearbook 2* (Milton Keynes: Open University Press), pp. 1–13.

Bamford, T. (1990), *The Future of Social Work* (London: Macmillan Education).

Barclay, P. (1982), *Social Workers: their Roles and Tasks* (London: Bedford Square Press).

Barrett, M. and McIntosh, M. (1985), 'Ethnocentrism and socialist-feminist theory', *Feminist Review* 20, pp. 23–48.

Bell, S. (1988), *When Salem came to the Boro: the True Story of the Cleveland Child Abuse Crisis* (London: Pan).

Birke, L., Himmelweit, S. and Vines, G. (1990), *Tomorrow's Child: Reproductive Technologies in the 90s* (London: Virago).
Brewer, C. and Lait, J. (1980), *Can Social Work Survive?* (London: Temple Smith).
Brook, E. and Davis, A. (1985), *Women, the Family and Social Work* (London: Tavistock).

Campbell, B. (1988), *Unofficial Secrets: Child Sexual Abuse: The Cleveland Case* (London: Virago).
CCETSW (1985), *Ethnic Minorities and Social Work Training*, Paper 21.1, October (London: CCETSW).
CCETSW (1986–89), *Data on Training and Reports on Applications* (London: CCETSW).
Challis, D. and Davies, B. (1986), *Case Management in Community Care* (Aldershot: Gower).
Channer, Y. and Parton, N. (1990), 'Racism, cultural relativism and child protection', in The Violence Against Children Study Group (eds), *Taking Child Abuse Seriously* (London: Unwin Hyman) pp. 105–20.
Clarke, J., Langan, M. and Lee, P. (1980), 'Social work: the conditions of crisis', in P. Carlen and M. Collison (eds), *Radical Issues in Criminology* (Oxford: Martin Robertson) pp 178–95.
Commission for Racial Equality (1983), *Children in Care* (London: CRE).
Coote, A., Harman, H. and Hewitt, P. (1990), *The Family Way*, Social Policy Paper 1 (London: Institute for Public Policy Research).
Currie, E. (12 July 1988) *Hansard*.

Dale, P. with Davies, M., Morrison, T. and Waters, J. (1986), *Dangerous Families: Assessment and Treatment of Child Abuse* (London: Tavistock).
Davis, A. and Brook, E. (1985), 'Women and social work', in E. Brook and A. Davis (eds), *Women, the Family and Social Work* (London: Tavistock) pp. 3–27.
Department of Health (1989), *The Children Act* (London: HMSO).
Department of Health (1989), *An Introduction to the Children Act* (London: HMSO).
Department of Health (1990), *Children Come First* Cmnd 1264 (London: HMSO).
Devlin, T. (6 July 1988) *Hansard*.
Dominelli, L. (1988), *Anti-Racist Social Work* (London: Macmillan).
Dutt, R. (1989), 'Griffiths really is a White Paper', *Social Work Today*, 23.

Elliot, F. Robertson (1986), *The Family: Change or Continuity* (London: Macmillan).

Family Policy Studies Centre (February 1988), *Young People at the Crossroads* (London: Family Policy Studies Centre).
Feminist Review (eds) (1988), *Family Secrets: Child Sexual Abuse*, *Feminist Review* 28.
Finch, J. (1988), 'Whose responsibility? Women and the future of family

care', in I. Allen, M. Wicks, J. Finch and D. Leet, *Informal Care Tomorrow* (London: PSI) pp. 22–31.
Finch, J. (1989), *Family Obligations and Social Change* (Cambridge: Polity Press).
Finch, J. (1990), 'The politics of community care in Britain', in C. Ungerson (ed.), *Gender and Caring: Work and Welfare in Britain and Scandinavia* (Hemel Hempstead: Harvester Wheatsheaf) pp. 34–58.
Foster, J. (1987), 'Women on the Wane', *Insight* 2, 50, pp. 14–15.
Frost, N. and Stein, M. (1989), *The Politics of Child Welfare* (Hemel Hempstead: Harvester Wheatsheaf).
Frost, N. and Stein, M. (1990), 'The politics of the Children Act', *Childright*, July/August, pp. 17–19.

Gardiner, D. (1985), *Ethnic Minorities and Social Work Training* Paper 21.1, October (London: CCETSW).
Gordon, L. (1986), 'Feminism and social control: the case of child abuse and neglect', in J. Mitchell and A. Oakley (eds), *What is Feminism?* (Oxford: Basil Blackwell) pp. 63–84.
Greenland, C. (1987), *Preventing CAN Deaths: An International Study of Deaths due to Child Abuse and Neglect* (London: Tavistock).
Griffiths, R. (1988), *Community Care: Agenda for Action* (London: HMSO).

Hall, S. (1989), *The Voluntary Sector Under Attack?* (London: IVAC).
Hallett, C. (1989), 'The gendered world of the social services department', in C. Hallett (ed.), *Women and Social Services Departments* (Hemel Hempstead: Harvester Wheatsheaf) pp. 1–43.
Henwood, M. (1990), *Community Care and Elderly People* (London: Family Policy Studies Centre).
Henwood, M., Rimmer, L. and Wicks, M. (1989), *Inside the Family: Changing Roles of Men and Women* (London: Family Policy Studies Centre).
HMSO (1989), *Caring for People: Community Care in the Next Decade and Beyond* Cmnd 849 (London: HMSO).
Home Office (1990), *Crime, Justice and Protecting the Public* Cmnd 965 (London: HMSO).
Howe, D. (1986), 'The segregation of women and their work in the personal social services', *Critical Social Policy*, 15, pp. 21–35.
Hughes, R. D. and Bhaduri, R. (1987), *Social Services for Ethnic Minorities and Race and Culture in Social Services Delivery* (Manchester: DHSS Social Services Inspectorate NW Region).

Jones, G. (1989), 'Women in social care: the invisible army', in Hallet 1989, pp. 132–54.

Kent, P., Pierson, J. and Thornton, B. (1990), 'Guide to the Children Act 1989', *Community Care* 19 April.
Kiernan, K. and Wicks, M. (1990), *Family Change and Future Policy* (London: Family Policy Provides Centre).
Knapp, M. (1989), 'Private and voluntary welfare' in M. McCarthy (ed.),

The New Politics of Welfare: an Agenda for the 1990s? (London: Macmillan) pp. 225–52.

LACSAB/ADSS (1989), *Survey of Social Services Employment 1988* (London: LACSAB Research Division and ADSS).

Land, H. (1978), 'Who cares for the family?' *Journal of Social Policy* 7, pp. 257–84.

Langan, M. (1985), 'The unitary approach: a feminist critique', in E. Brook and A. Davis 1985, pp. 3–27.

Langan, M. (1988), 'Women under Thatcherism', in Alcock and Lee 1988, pp. 65–71.

Langan, M. (1990), 'Comunity care in the 1990s', *Critical Social Policy*, 29, pp. 58–70.

Langan, M. and Lee, P. (1989), 'Whatever happened to radical work?' in M. Langan and P. Lee (eds), *Radical Social Work Today* (London: Unwin Hyman) pp. 1–18.

Leonard, P. (1982), 'Review of "the essential social worker": a guide to positive practice', *Critical Social Policy*, 1, 3, pp. 78–80.

London Borough of Brent (1985), *A Child in Trust: Report of the panel of inquiry investigating the circumstances surrounding the death of Jasmine Beckford* (London Borough of Brent).

London Borough of Greenwich (1987), *A Child in Mind: Protection of Children in a Responsible Society. Report of the commission of inquiry into the circumstances surrounding the death of Kimberley Carlile* (London Borough of Greenwich).

London Borough of Lambeth (1987), *Whose Child? The report of the panel appointed to inquire into the death of Tyra Henry* (London Borough of Lambeth).

McCarthy, M. (ed.) (1989), *The New Politics of Welfare: an Agenda for the 1990s?* (London: Macmillan).

McCarthy, M. (1989), 'Personal social services', in McCarthy 1989, pp. 22–52.

NALGO (1989), *Social Work in Crisis: A Study of Conditions in six Local Authorities* (London: NALGO).

NCVO (1989), *Critical Issues for Black and Ethnic Minority Groups, Contracts for Care* (London: NCVO).

Parker, G. (1990), *With Due Care and Attention* (London: Family Policy Studies Centre).

Parton, C. (1990), 'Women, gender oppression and child abuse', in The Violence Against Children Study Group 1990, pp. 41–62.

Parton, C. and Parton, N. (1989), 'Child protection, the law and dangerousness', in O. Stevenson (ed.), *Child Abuse: Professional Practice and Public Policy* (Hemel Hempstead: Harvester Wheatsheaf) pp. 54–73.

Parton, N. (1991), *Governing the Family: Child Care, Child Protection and the State* (London: Macmillan).

Pascall, G. (1986), *Social Policy: A Feminist Analysis* (London: Tavistock).

Pinker, R. (1985), 'Family services', in R. Berthoud (ed.), *Challenges to Social Policy* (London: PSI) pp. 72–101.
Pinker, R. (nd), 'Planning the mixed economy of care', unpublished paper.
Popplestone, R. (1980), 'Top jobs for women: are the cards stacked against them?', *Social Work Today* 12, 4, pp. 12–15.

Redding, D. (1989), 'Deregulating day care', *Community Care*, 15 June.
Rooney, B. (1982), 'Black social workers in white departments', in J. Cheetham (ed.), *Social Work and Ethnicity* (London: NISW/George Allen and Unwin) pp. 184–96.
Rooney, B. (1987), *Racism and Resistance to Change: A Study of the Black Social Workers' Project, Liverpool Social Services Department 1975–1985* (Liverpool: Department of Sociology, University of Liverpool).
Roys, P. (1988), 'Social Services' in A. Bhat, R. Carr-Hill and S. Ohri (eds), *Britain's Black Population: A New Perspective* 2nd Edition (Aldershot: Gower) pp. 208–36.

Smart, C. (1987), 'Securing the family? rhetoric and policy in the field of social security', in M. Loney *et al.* (eds), *The State or the Market* (London: Sage) pp. 99–114.
Smart, C. (1989), *Feminism and the Power of Law* (London: Routledge).
Smith, D. (nd), *From Seebohm to Barclay: the Changing Political Nature of the Organisation of Social Work* Discussion paper (Manchester: Department of Social Administration, University of Manchester).

Thatcher, M. (1990), 'The Pankhurst Lecture, 17 July 1990', *The Guardian* 18 July.
Thompson, C. (1989), *Should Voluntary Organisations Provide More Services?* Community Care Project, Contracts for Care 2 (London: NCVO).

Ungerson, C. (ed.) (1990), *Gender and Caring: Work and Welfare in Britain and Scandinavia* (Hemel Hempstead: Harvester Wheatsheaf).
Ungerson, C. (1990), 'The language of care: crossing the boundaries' in Ungerson (ed.) 1990, pp. 8–33.

Violence Against Children Study Group (eds) (1990), *Taking Child Abuse Seriously* (London: Unwin Hyman).

Walker, A. (1984), 'The political economy of privatisation', in J. LeGrand and R. Robinson (eds), *Privatisation and the Welfare State* (London: George Allen and Unwin) pp. 19–44.
Weeks, J. (1985), *Sexuality and its Discontents: Meanings, Myths and Modern Sexualities* (London: Routledge).
Wicks, M. (1990), 'The battle for the family', *Marxism Today*, August, pp. 28–33.
Wilson, E. (1977), *Women and the Welfare State* (London: Tavistock).

5 *Feminism, managerialism and performance measurement*

Carol Lupton

Introduction

While we must beware of attributing a greater degree of coherence to government philosophies than their practical expression would warrant, two central political themes have been of particular relevance to the development of personal social services over the past decade. The first derives from the wider attempt to restructure the welfare state: to stimulate a more central role for the voluntary and private sectors and to encourage a greater degree of individual rather than state reliance. Successive Conservative administrations have demonstrated a strong ideological distaste for large, monolithic bureaucracies which they believe deny choice and limit innovation, and have made clear their admiration for the competitive market. Their consistent failure to distinguish between the role of the organized voluntary sector on the one hand and informal 'voluntary effort' on the other moreover reveals a determination to underpin the public provision of social care with a widespread reliance on informal care networks. This shift in the balance of care has been legitimated by the political drive to re-establish the centrality of the family in social life.

The second major theme of relevance to this chapter is the systematic attempt by central government to extend its control over the expenditure of local authorities. The lack of effective mechanisms for enabling central political control over the activities of local authorities has long been considered problematic by the Conservatives. The 1982 Select Committee on Social Services complained that there were 'no sophisticated indicators for central government to make serious assessments of local authority service provision' (Great Britain, Parliament 1982: 306–1 p. 39, para. 105). The 1980s witnessed an increasingly determined series of attempts – through the 1980 Local Government, Planning and Land Act and the subsequent 1984 Rates Act in particular – to reduce and restructure the spending of local government.

Both tendencies – the general restructuring of welfare and the tightened control of the local authorities – have made an impact on the role of the local authorities in the provision of personal social services. The publication in 1989 of the White Paper *Caring for People* (HMSO 1989) outlining the Conservative government's proposals for the reorganization of community care services, represents the explicit culmination of both tendencies. The new role of the local authorities as the 'broker' or 'ring-holder' of community care services, responsible for coordinating and purchasing non-health care from an increasingly pluriform care market, may signal the end of their role as mainstream providers of social care. The relucant acceptance by the government of the need to give local authorities this responsibility is however accompanied by a determination to increase their financial and political accountability. The Conservatives have publically expressed their reservations about the ability of these organizations to undertake their new role, and the White Paper reveals the government's intention to take new powers to inspect local authorities' community care plans and to ensure that these are developed in close conjunction with national objectives and priorities (HMSO 1989: 41, para 5.2).

The government believes that the lack of cost-effectiveness on the part of public health and welfare organizations stems in large part from the dominance of a backward-looking 'service-orientated' managerial practice. If local authorities are to adapt to the new climate of 'care purchasing', it insists, they will need to develop a more 'business-like' organizational culture. Unlike the health service however, where central government has been able to impose new managerial styles directly, changes to local government's organizational culture have had to be effected more indirectly. The establishment of the Audit Commission in 1983 and the reformulation in 1985 of the Social Services Inspectorate aimed to improve the economy, efficiency and effectiveness of local authorities' service provision. Their operation increased the possibilities of stimulating a new, more entrepreneurial managerialism within local authority social services departments. As Kelly has argued: 'The Audit Commission has been the major visible institutional manifestation of the government's desire to promote the new managerialism within local government' (Kelly 1989: 3).

Central to the new managerial approach is the more effective production and use of knowledge within the organization. One of the main concerns of the Griffiths report on the provision of community care was the general inadequacy of social services departments' internal information systems. The report's admonishment that their: 'present lack of refined information systems . . . would plunge most organisations in the private sector into quick and merciful liquidation' (HMSO 1989: viii, para 28) placed the issue of the organizational information-base high on political and managerial agendas. It became increasingly recognized that good internal information systems were essential if departments were to identify and review the results of their 'performance' more systematically – a central prerequisite for a more cost-effective managerial approach. In *Caring for People* the government warned that local authority social services departments would be charged with establishing adequate mechanisms for measuring their performance (HMSO 1989: 43, para 5.14). The government would in turn take steps to ensure that this performance was measured against 'national objectives' (HMSO 1989: 41, para 5.2).

This chapter examines the characteristics of the new managerialism within social services departments from a feminist perspective. The impact of the new managerialist culture on the quality of organizational knowledge is explored and specific attention paid to the development of mechanisms for performance measurement. It argues that pressures for greater accountability represent potentially a positive force for change within social services departments. A more public evaluation of performance is a necessary precondition of an improved quality of service provision, particularly with the emergence of a more pluriform care market. However we need to examine closely the particular measures of performance being developed within social services departments, and assess the values and assumptions which underlie them. What aspects of organizational activity will they describe, and what kind of organizational 'accountability' will they deliver? What is the quality of the knowledge on which they are based and will they be informed by the views of clients and service users? Most importantly, will they result in an improved quality of service provision and increase social services departments' ability to identify and overcome the effects of systematic sex, race and class discrimination? This chapter will attempt to provide some answers to these central questions.

The knowledge-base as a site for feminist struggle?

The knowledge-base of any social services department is developed in a number of ways: by its awareness of and receptivity to political and ideological debates at a national level; by the work of academic researchers and policy analysts both nationally and locally; by the accumulated skills and expertise of the department's staff, and thus by the quality of in-house or externally based training; by the intellectual gatekeeping of social work's professional body; and finally by the research and information gathering activity of that department itself (and its counterparts elsewhere). It is this last area of knowledge-generation which is the specific concern of this chapter.

Although such internal knowledge is intimately related to wider knowledges – in so far as these will inform the parameters of what is considered relevant and useful – it is distinguishable by its focus on the specific activities, resources and context of the organization itself. This internally generated knowledge plays a central role in informing both the general organizational ethos or culture of the department, as well as its specific policies and practices. In particular, and of central importance to the argument of this chapter, it informs crucial policy decisions concerning both the distribution of resources and the objectives of social work practice. As such, the organizational knowledge-base represents a central site for feminist and anti-racist political and ideological struggle.

The generation of knowledge has both a radical and a reactionary potential: it can be a force for progressive change or a means of legitimating and maintaining an oppressive status quo. In the case of the official collection of race statistics, for example, the government has argued that more detailed knowledge about the lives of black and minority ethnic people will enable it to provide better resources and services and formulate more effective strategies for overcoming discrimination. The Commission for Racial Equality developed similar arguments in pushing for the inclusion of a race and ethnic origin question in the 1981 census (CRE 1980). Clearly, the effective monitoring of equal opportunities policies requires the careful collection of data concerning the operation of sex or race discrimination. On the other hand the gathering of data, particularly around issues of policing and immigration, can serve to reinforce stereotypes and prejudices about black people, and provide legitimation to those who are interested in extending rather than confronting the operation of racial discrimination (Ohri 1988).

As the above debate reveals, the generation of social data is not a neutral 'technical' process; rather it is affected by the dominant power relations which structure the specific context of its collection and use. Typically it is those with power who gather information about those without power: 'The eyes of sociologists, with few but honorable exceptions, have been turned downwards, and their palms upwards' (Nicolaus 1972: 39), and it is those with power who have the greatest control over the use to which this information is put. In societies which are structured by race, sex and class discrimination, the nature and use of 'official' social data will not necessarily reflect the interests of those who are black, female and poor.

It is, moreover, not only the generation and use of social knowledge which is value-laden, but also the way in which that knowledge is obtained. As feminist and black critiques have demonstrated, both what is known (the object of scientific study) and the way in which it is known (the methods of scientific study) have been infected by the values and assumptions of the white middle-class males who have dominated mainstream scientific practice. Despite its posturings of value freedom and objectivity, both the process and product of scientific activity have reflected the fact that it has been dominated by 'a particular sub-set of the human race' (Fox-Keller 1985: 7). Indeed, the central notion of 'objectivity' itself, in so far as it is defined as the antithesis of subjective experience, encapsulates male meanings and male ways of relating to the world: 'Science is cold, hard, impersonal, "objective", women, by contrast, are warm, soft, emotional, "subjective" ' (Fee 1983: 13).

One of the central manifestations of a masculinized institutional knowledge-base is the systematic absence of women as a category of knowledge. This invisibility typically originates from, and is compounded by, sex-blind or gender-biased research and information-gathering techniques. Sex-blindness occurs most commonly when the process of data collection simply ignores the sex of the respondent or client as a relevant variable. Without so 'stratifying' the data, however, it is impossible for researchers or policy-makers to assess whether the needs and experiences of women clients are any different from those of male clients, and whether a different kind of service or social work response is consequently needed. The sex-related inequalities in domiciliary service provision revealed in studies by Hunt (1970) and others, for example, would remain unidentified within a sex-blind institutional data base. These methodological sins of omission are compounded when the absence of sex as an organizing category is accompanied by the absence of the categories of race or class. Crucial information concerning the specific needs or experiences of black or working-class women and girls, such as their statistically disproportionate tendency to suffer the controlling and coercive practices of statutory agencies (CRE 1983; DHSS 1984; Harrison *et al.* 1984), may in this way remain concealed.

Gender-bias (methodological androcentrism) occurs when data gathered predominantly on the basis of male experience or needs are presented as applying equally to all clients, male or female. Studies of the problem-drinker or the juvenile offender are typically of this nature, with services being centrally structured around male patterns of behaviour, and the issue of whether women drinkers or young female offenders have significantly different needs in respect of service provision being ignored (Bennett 1982; Hudson 1988). Gender-bias also occurs when the process of data gathering is affected by the operation of implicit assumptions about the different forms of behaviour appropriate to men and women. Such assumptions, as Eichler (1988) has so painstakingly documented, can seriously distort all stages of the generation of knowledge, from the initial conceptualization of the problem to be studied, to the analysis and interpretation of the 'findings'. Again the ability of official statistics to mystify and misinform is intensified when gender-biased data collection is overlain by racist or class-based assumptions.

The central problem with the quality of the knowledge so generated (apart from its lack of scientific rigour and 'objectivity') is that the invisibility of women as a category of knowledge typically results in the invisibility of women from the policy considerations of social services departments. The absence of women as 'inputs' to the policy process almost inevitably entails their subsequent absence in policy 'outputs'. Crucial decisions about who gets what are thus uninformed by knowledge of the specific needs and experiences of different groups of women. As a result of its partial and value-laden categorizations, the effect of a sex-blind and gender-biased knowledge system can be not only to ignore, but also to reinforce, the reality of the oppression suffered by black, white and working-class women.

Where women are in a very real sense hidden from the policy process, the production of 'official' knowledge about the specific experiences and needs of women and girls may have a radical potential. While it is impossible to ensure that the collection of comprehensive public data concerning the nature and extent of discrimination in service provision will tilt the hand of service providers, we can be very certain that the opposite is true: the continued lack of such data will serve only to perpetuate the inattention which policy-makers currently give such issues. As the role of local authority social services departments changes, their knowledge infrastructures will become more critical in affecting the distribution of resources in a more diversified care market. In this context it is essential that the androcentric and ethnocentric nature of much organizational 'knowledge' is identified, and confronted with more methodologically rigorous data which reveal the particular experiences and needs of black and white female clients.

The new managerialism

In order to assess the tendencies affecting the quality of knowledge generated within social services departments, we need to explore the emergent features of what has been termed the 'new managerialist' approach. Although we should acknowledge the difficulty of generalizing about a situation characterized by a variety of practices, it is possible to identify some central, ideal-typical features of this new managerialism. The first is a move away from the traditional individualized style of leadership and concern with the internal processes, to a corporate style managerial practice centring on the external performance of the organization. Accompanying this more outward-directed tendency is the emergence of a strategic, goal-setting managerial style. The result being not so much an alternative to the old bureaucratic managerial approach as an attempt to 'pep it up with an injection of business spirit' (Hadley 1986: 1).

The development of a more professional managerialism demands new and different kinds of skills on the part of senior managers. They must be able to build and sustain the 'strategic vision of the organisation' (Etherington 1989a: 20) and ensure that it is equipped to implement this vision effectively. They will need to be highly specific about objectives and able to 'define these in behaviourable and measurable terms' (Bamford 1982: 178). Required to move from 'demand scarcity' planning to a more cost-led 'supply planning' approach, the new managers must be able to position the organization to take maximum advantage of its changing environment. They must be 'skilled in organisational design and willing to experiment with structural change' (Etherington 1989a: 20). Increasingly, they will need to respond appropriately 'to the calls for greater effectiveness and demonstrations of the cost-benefit of social work intervention' (Bamford 1982: 178).

Clearly, the skills required of this ideal-typical new manager are considerable; we can surmise that the bulk of current senior management within social services departments only imperfectly and probably rather hesitantly lives up to such expectations. Nevertheless the general tenets of the new managerial theories are achieving an increased currency. What are the central characteristics of those who may be required or eager to embrace them?

The first central feature of the new managers is that they are likely to be overwhelmingly male. The existence of organizational 'gender pyramids' within social services departments, where a small number of males dominate the apex and a large number of women constitute the base, has by now been well established. The sharp decline of women in senior positions following the 1971 reorganization of departments has been extended more incrementally with each successive reorganization (Popplestone 1980; Foster 1987). More recent organizational 'slimming and trimming' – in particular the discontinuation of many deputy directorships – has consolidated the sexual division of labour within departments. Currently less than 10 per cent of directors are women, and there is evidence that departments headed by women are significantly smaller than those led by men (Foster 1987).

The second central characteristic of the new manager is that he (*sic*) will almost certainly be white. The strength of the colour-blind approach is such that it is difficult to get accurate data on the proportion of black staff employed at various levels within local authority social services departments. Research conducted by a joint ADSS/CRE working party in the late 1970s found that 90 per cent of the departments surveyed kept no systematic records on the ethnic composition of their staff. (Three quarters kept no records on the ethnic origin of clients.) (Cheetham *et al.* 1981). What data exist indicate that the number of black senior staff is low: an SSI survey of 17 departments in the north west of the country found only three black staff at principal officer level or above (Hughes and Bhaduri 1990). The survey did not reveal the sex of these staff, but it is clear that black women aspiring to senior management posts have to face a double barrier. The difficulties of succeeding as a woman within a masculinist organizational culture will be compounded by the problems of overcoming racist stereotyping and practice. The heightened competitiveness of the new managerialist culture is not likely to diminish the size or the durability of the hurdles faced by black people seeking managerial positions.

The third feature of the new managers is their commitment to the pursuit of a 'career ideal' rather than to the development of a 'service ideal'. In this they are likely to differ from more traditional managers, whether male or female. In a recent study, Foster (1988a) identifies the growing phenomenon of 'department hopping' on the part of upwardly mobile male staff. In the search for career advancement, these men move rapidly from one department to another, often leaving after a process of restructuring which they themselves have initiated. Typically, they are more likely to achieve promotion as successful external candidates than as promoted internal ones. In addition to being almost always male, these new managers are relatively young: 'Age at first directorship appears to be one of the strongest predictive factors in identifying a prospective department hopper' (Foster 1988a: 20). Rather than the values of continuity of service and familiarity with the historical and local context of the department, the attributes being sought in the new managers appear to be: 'youth, masculinity and mobility' (Foster 1988a: 21).

Although not deriving simply from the numerical dominance of men within senior management, recent years have witnessed an increased masculinization of the managerial process which may in turn enhance the tendency to a greater physical male dominance. To the extent that success depends on the 'seemingly relentless pursuit of salary and status' (Foster 1988b: 12) women may be increasingly reluctant to apply for managerial positions. Women are more likely to achieve seniority in departments where they have worked for considerable lengths of time, and to achieve that seniority at a later age (Foster 1988b). They may, moreover, be more likely than their male colleagues to remain committed to the service ideal. Studies by Cooper and Davidson (1982) and Eley (1987) indicate that women in senior managerial positions view their roles and responsibilities differently from male managers. Whereas men typically value the bureaucratic requirements of the job, women managers emphasize the more 'supportive, caring part of the job' (Eley 1987: 13). While it is important to avoid an essentialist reading of the above studies, and to resist the notion that women are somehow inherently predisposed to more expressive and caring ways of working, it is clear that the more explicitly masculinized culture of the new managerialism may be an increasingly difficult environment for many women to work effectively within.

Managerialism and the new knowledge

Effective and efficient management requires the best possible available knowledge, yet there are tendencies within the new managerialism which may have serious consequences for the quality of the organizational knowledge-base. The increased fine-tuning of knowledge production to the specific and often short-term objectives of policy-makers may result in the prioritization of a certain kind of knowledge which is limited in both reliability and scope. The current uneasy role of research within social services departments may be instructive here.

Much has been written about the under-utilization of research in social services departments (Trow 1984; Booth 1986). Booth, among others, lays the blame for the policy-makers' lack of interest squarely on the shoulders of researchers themselves, particularly those who are based in academic institutions. Researchers, he argues, have simply 'failed to deliver the goods' (Booth 1986: 15): they have not learned to adapt to the new political environment surrounding social services departments, and as a result have not been able to give the policy-makers what they want.

Booth contends that the requirements for good academic research are not the same as those for policy-relevant research: 'These different tasks call for a different science' (Booth 1986: 16). In particular, he argues, academics must learn to make a 'judicious trade-off' between the requirements of intellectual rigour and those of policy relevance. The major characteristic of policy-relevant research is not its reliability or its validity, but its utility (Booth 1986: 17) and the main way to ensure utility is to accept the objectives of the policy-maker as guides for the research process. Others have argued similarly that the distinguishing characteristic of the policy analyst as opposed to the academic researcher is that 'He or she is trained, indeed required, to see and formulate problems from the perspectives not of the academic disciplines, but of the decision maker' (Trow 1984).

The problem with this kind of argument is that it renders the quality of knowledge generated within social services departments conditional on the intellectual scope and perspicacity of the policy-makers. As Booth himself points out: 'Research that outstrips their comprehension is unlikely to receive their backing' (Booth 1986: 18). Such a condition, however, is likely to operate as a central constraint over the range of internally generated knowledge. Thus Weiss and Bucuvalas (1980) contend that as well as imposing a utility test, decision-makers apply a 'truth' test to all available data: the 'truth' being defined in terms of the extent to which new findings conform to already-held beliefs and prior understandings. The effect of this method of 'successive limited comparisons' (Lindblom 1959) may be the emergence of an inherently conservative institutional knowledge-base. Research which involves areas outside the already marked-up 'information windows' is simply seen as irrelevant. Anything that seeks to reveal or question the values underlying the decisions of policy-makers may be seen as a positive 'disutility'.

To the extent that knowledge is redefined as a strategic organizational input, this instrumentalist approach to knowledge is likely to be exacerbated within the new managerialism. Thus we are told that an organization: 'needs an information strategy, as much as it needs a financial strategy, a strategy for its capital assets and a strategy for its human resources' (Fletcher 1988: 17). Valued only as a strategic input, however, the integrity of knowledge can be severely impaired. As knowledge becomes a weapon in the cut and thrust of policy negotiation, its utility becomes inextricably linked to its ability to convince. In the context of a masculinized organizational culture, knowledge may be at its most convincing when it is presented as 'hard', as 'objective' and unequivocal 'facts'.

The spurious distinction between 'objective' and 'subjective' knowledge becomes confused with the distinction between 'qualitative' and 'quantitative' data. Encouraged by the rapid computerization of management information systems, preference is more readily given to the apparent certainties and often deceptive truths of data which have been heavily quantified. Knowledge inputs are considered to be of optimal utility when they come in small, preferably discrete, bite- (or byte-) sized pieces. The more the complexity of human interaction is simplified, the better it may be seen to 'fit' the requirements of departments subject to external pressures to monitor and measure their performance. One central effect of this tendency to value easily quantifiable information inputs has been an increased disjunction between the activity of gathering information and the process of doing research. Montgomery (1988) anticipates that the result will be the diminution of the research role and its transmutation into a more administrative function, supporting and servicing the development of the new technology. Without significant counterbalancing tendencies, the nineties could witness the demise of the researcher and the emergence of the new 'information technocrat' (Barritt 1987).

Although at present the emergence of these tendencies is partial and uneven, they signal an increased marginality for feminist thought and practice within social services departments. The more extensive the masculinization of the departments' organizational cultures under the impact of the new managerialism, the more overtly masculinized will be the knowledge systems generated. For the newly entrepreneurial manager in pursuit of 'strategic opportunism', it is likely that feminist-inspired research will be seen to deliver the wrong kind of knowledge, collected in the wrong kind of way, about the wrong kinds of things.

The focus of feminist research on areas whose importance is typically resisted by policy-makers has not endeared it to those who control the production of knowledge within social services departments. Its epistemologies, moreover, may seek to prioritize a very different kind of knowledge, generated in very different ways, from that which appears so neatly to fit the needs of the policy process. The prejudices that many senior decision-takers hold about feminist research – the subjective and irrelevant, pursued by the angry and emotional – may be reinforced if the more general trend to devalue the production of longer-term, more theoretically informed research (whether qualitative or quantitative) achieves dominance. The ability of feminists to undertake research within and into social services departments may as a result be doubly circumscribed.

Performance indicators – a case in point?

The history of performance measurement within social services departments is relatively brief. The development of forward planning within the personal social services (the LAPS, or Local Authority Planning Statements) petered out in the late 1970s as a result of a lack of adequate data (Miller 1986), and the Rayner investigation in the early 1980s reduced the volume of data collected on social services departments by the then DHSS. Since the mid-1980s, however, there has been a series of attempts to establish national measures of performance which enable inter-authority comparison of service provision. The Audit Commission's attempt to measure local authority 'profiles' against other local authorities in the same 'family' (that family being identified on the basis of census data) has been followed more recently by the Social Services Inspectorate's (SSI) 'Key Indicators' (KI) initiative.

First released in December 1988 as a demonstration package, the KI project attempted to bring together data from a wide range of sources – including financial data from the Chartered Institute of Public Finance and Accountancy (CIPFA), DSS staffing and activity returns, DOE rate fund accounts and OPCS population estimates – to provide 'a powerful analytical tool kit' (Warburton 1989a: 6) for assessing the performance of social services departments. As with the Audit Commission's local profiles, the objective was to discover the norm and to identify those local authorities which significantly deviate – 'the outliers'. The eventual aim was to establish an 'expert system' providing standardized reports on all individual departments: 'an initial description and commentary on local authority services based on broad brush national data' (Warburton 1989b: 23).

The central problem with the indicator package is the limited and distorted nature of the data it utilizes. Thus Hardingham (1986), Miller (1986), and others, have indicated how, as a result either of the inadequacy of individual departments' internal information systems and/or of the variation in their interpretation of identical categories, the data underlying the indicators are of poor or variable quality. Problems with the conceptual adequacy of the data, however, are not only one way; there is growing evidence that many social services departments are forced to make misleading recordings because they are unable to find the appropriate category on the official data collection forms (Hardingham 1986). Studies by Knapp (1987) and others, moreoever, have revealed the extent to which calculations concerning the relative cost of different areas of service provision are often made on an entirely erroneous basis, with the result that inter-departmental comparisons are crude and misleading. An independent field study carried out in 1989 as part of the KI initiative indeed found many data items unreliable as a basis for inter-agency comparison (Warburton 1989c).

Two of the most serious inadequacies of the data comprising the indicator package are their androcentrism and ethnocentrism; the apparent value neutrality of the indicators is belied by their sex and race-blindness. Although the CIPFA actuals and the Audit Commission's profiles make use of data structured by client group and age, no information is systematically collected on service provision by sex or race of client.

Some attempt has been made recently by the SSI to increase the race sensitivity of its data collection activities. Pearson argues that proposals currently being put into effect should mean the 'end of colour blind inspections and reports' (Pearson 1989: 14). He concedes, however, that it may be 'some time' before the Inspectorate is able to address issues of race and culture with the same authority it brings to other subjects. Ironically, the attempt by the SSI to draw up a programme of inspection visits to social services departments to examine 'how they were responding to a multi-racial society' highlighted the fact that the only black employees of the SSI were in administrative and clerical posts. Acknowledging that it would 'lack credibility' if its inspections were carried out by an exclusively white group of inspectors, the SSI coopted black colleagues from outside agencies to act as consultants.

It is not in any way to belittle the importance of such developments to note the irony of the fact that the lack of black inspectors was not seen to reduce the credibility of the Inspectorate in pursuance of its mainstream activities. It is also worth noting that none of the same sensitivity is evident in respect of the SSI's attitude towards sex inequality. There appears to be little concern with the credibility of a largely male Inspectorate assessing the effectiveness of services provided to predominantly female clients by a mainly female body of social care and social work staff. In its attempt to assist local authorities to develop services which are 'accessible and relevant to all sections of the community' the Inspectorate apparently fails to acknowledge women and girls as an identifiable section of that community (Pearson 1989: 15).

Thus, for example, data on services for mentally ill people examine only the number (and cost per head) of training centres, sheltered employment and day care places provided for the client group taken as a whole. We have no way of monitoring the extent to which these services are available equally to male and female, black and white clients. Again, Audit data on children in care examine only age and the different forms of placement as a percentage of the total in-care population. Yet evidence suggests significant sex- and race-related differences in both placements and outcomes (CRE 1983; Lupton 1985). It is clear that as a mechanism for assessing and comparing organizational performance such statistical data are seriously inadequate.

There is evidence too that a more active gender bias undermines the validity of the data comprising the indicators. For example, assessments of the relative expenditure of different services provided by social services departments typically fail to cost adequately all components of the care provided. Although making the assumption (itself gender-laden) that elderly clients living in sheltered housing receive substantial amounts of informal support from relatives or friends, the Audit Guide makes no attempt to assess the reality of that assumption, nor to include the costs of such care in comparative cost calculations (Miller 1986). Yet, as has by now been well established, the comparative cheapness of community care alternatives for many client groups is achieved only by ignoring the very considerable costs borne by their predominantly female carers. Again, we find that the nature of the knowledge informing the indicators is partial and misleading.

A further, related, problem with the indicator data is their concentration on service 'inputs' – cost of services, number of staff, number of clients and so on – at the expense of any similarly detailed examination of 'outcomes' or impact of the services provided. Only limited assessment of the effectiveness of services will thus be possible at a national level. We will know how many residential homes for elderly people are provided by a local authority, for example, how much they cost and how many staff work in them, but little if anything about the quality of those homes, the suitability of their location, the accessibility of the services they provide and, most importantly, the experience of the elderly people living within them. These more qualitative forms of data will be left for local authorities to collect for themselves: 'largely due to the methodological difficulties of establishing and quantifying universally valid and reliable outcome measures in the field of social services' (Warburton 1989a: 16).

The KI package was not designed to substitute for social services departments' own internal evaluations; these, it was believed, would be needed to contextualize and elaborate the indicator information. The SSI thus takes great pains to emphasize that the KI data cannot be taken as definitive measures of performance in themselves, but should rather be used to trigger more questions and the collection of more data. Their value rests 'on building an agenda of questions and starting points for more detailed studies involving local data' (Warburton 1989b: 23). Yet it is likely that these more detailed local data, precisely because they are more difficult to collect, will be less readily sought by the new-style managers. Hardingham's survey (1986) of managers' responses to the Audit Commission's profiles indicates that many feel their proper interpretation represents an onerous task. The evidence of the NHS indicates that, once established professional and organizational energies concentrate on improving the technical adequacy of existing indicators, rather than on expanding their range and scope. In particular, indicators of effectiveness which have to do with the more potentially politically embarrassing concepts of equity or consumer voice are typically eschewed in favour of 'the more neutral, technical sounding indicators such as cost per inpatient case' (Pollitt 1986: 21).

The main danger with the development of centrally collected statistical indicators is that, in the absence of more locally specific, evaluative data, they will be used by default as the basis for assessing the performance of individual social services departments. Thus Warburton concedes the possibility that some people may too readily equate a high or a low performance 'score' (PI value) with good or bad practice on the part of the department concerned (Warburton 1989b). Despite all the caveats, as we have seen, the assumption underlying the production of the indicators is that social services departments will use them to compare their performance and adjust it if necessary (James 1987). The very attractiveness of the indicators to the government is their function as an effective means of increasing central control over the departments and of ensuring a greater degree of uniformity in their service provision. In so far as they represent a mechanism for improving the accountability of social services departments, it is clear that the nature of this accountability will be cost- rather than need-related, and upward rather than downward in its line of vision.

Conclusion

This chapter has highlighted the more problematic tendencies within the emergent new managerialism. It should be acknowledged, however, that within the complex reality of any one individual social services department there will be limits on the extent to which any of these tendencies is fully played out in practice. Indeed, it is precisely the argument of this chapter that these issues are a vital area for political negotiation and struggle. The resistance of some senior managers, male and female, to the worst excesses of entrepreneurial managerialism, and the continued commitment of many managers and social workers to good quality practice and provision, will represent significant checks over the more extreme consequences of these developments. Nevertheless, no one concerned with the future of publicly provided personal social services can afford to ignore the rise of the new managerialism, nor the strength of the external pressures encouraging its progress.

Concentration on the more worrying implications of external pressures for greater efficiency and accountability should not blind us to their more progressive possibilities. In a context of uncertain and limited financial resources it is crucial that social services departments develop better (more publicly accessible) mechanisms for monitoring the effectiveness and equity of the services they provide. Such mechanisms will be all the more important given the changing balance of care, with social services departments increasingly sub-contracting the provision of services to those whose activities may be subject to only minimal public scrutiny. In this context the radical potential of increased concerns with performance measurement should be identified and exploited.

It is the argument of this chapter, however, that many of the measures of performance currently being developed both nationally and locally are antithetical to the aim of assuring an improved quality of local authority personal social services. The assessment of organizational performance within a welfare context must involve more than the collection and statistical manipulation of (often ill-assorted) descriptive activity indicators. Rather, it needs the best possible quality of information gathered by the widest possible range of methodological techniques. Crucially, it requires that systematic assessment of the outcome of service provision or social work intervention is made, and that in this assessment the evaluations of a number of different 'stake-holders' – particularly those of the users of a service – are taken into account. Above all, if local authorities are to monitor and implement the equal opportunities policies that most now profess, they must develop performance indicators which are sensitive to the effects of sex, race and class discrimination.

Evidence suggests that the priorities and preoccupations of cost-effective management may make the internal generation of good quality, user-relevant performance measures less likely in future years. The general tendency to downgrade the role of evaluative research within social service departments in favour of more limited information inputs, fine-tuned to the specific short-term requirements of policy-makers, may not provide the intellectual preconditions for a rigorous internal assessment of organizational performance. To the extent that the new entrepreneurial approach encourages concerns with the 'utility' of information over its validity or reliability, the poorer will be the quality of the knowledge which informs and underpins organizational policy and practice. In particular, the more masculinized the new managerial culture is, and the more obsessed it becomes with concerns of economy over those of effectiveness, the more insensitive its information systems are likely to be to the specific and general effects of sex, race and class oppression. Under these conditions the radical potential of performance assessment is unlikely to be fulfilled.

In this context the efforts of the national Social Services Research Group (SSRG) to devise a body of more wide-ranging and complex indicators to complement the work on the key indicators package is to be welcomed. Concerned initially about the 'inappropriate and incomplete' measures of performance being used by the Audit Commission in its value for money studies, some members of this group have argued the need for the development of more sophisticated and evaluative measures of performance which utilize a greater range and variety of data, both qualitative and quantitative. The generation of 'indicators', they argue, should be seen as only one element of a more wide-ranging strategy of performance measurement. This measurement should involve the collection of information about the experience of service users, representing thus 'a coherent collection of information on aspects of services provided and about those needing, seeking or receiving them' (Barnes and Miller 1988: 1).

The approach of the SSRG however (to which this chapter cannot do justice) may beg the vital question of whether the attraction of the key indicators to the government stems precisely from their current limited nature – from the fact that they collect certain kinds of information in certain kinds of ways. The political usefulness of the indicators is not unrelated to the fact that they are relatively quick and easy to produce, and enable some form of comparison – albeit rough and ready – by which to force 'rogue' departments into line. The SSRG may also be rather optimistic about the extent to which financially hard-pressed social services departments will be prepared (or able) to devote extra resources to the collection of more detailed evaluative data. In particular, the SSRG initiative may underestimate the extent to which the current nature of the indicators is inextricably bound up with some of the more problematic tendencies of the new managerialism. As such the proposal to 'add on' more user-friendly indicators may fail to recognize the deep-seated nature of the problem. As Barritt has argued, few of the changes required to ensure proper accountability are purely 'technical', but rather demand 'substantial changes in organisational behaviour' (Barritt 1987: 2).

Nevertheless, those concerned to increase the accountability of social services departments to service users must take account of the development and growing centrality of the key indicators approach. It cannot simply be ignored. Resistance to its influence, in its current form, may need to develop on two related fronts. The partial and misleading nature of the data underlying the indicators – in particular their insensitivity to issues of gender, race and class – must be systematically and publicly revealed. Individual departments must be pressed to develop more sophisticated measures of performance which emphasize the central relationship between service provision and user satisfaction. At the same time, it may be necessary to challenge the values and assumptions which underpin the performance indicators. This may mean confronting the more problematic tendencies of the new managerialist organizational culture. Thus, in addition to improving the mechanisms providing a department's self-assessment, we may need to push for a re-definition of its central organizational goals and objectives. This may be a tall order, but it is one in which all those committed to the more responsive and equitable provision of personal social services should have a vested interest.

References

Bamford, T. (1982), *Managing Social Work* (London: Tavistock).

Barnes, M. and Miller, N. (1988), 'Performance measurement in the personal social services', *Research, Policy and Planning* 6, 2, pp. 1–47.

Barnes, M. and Wilson, T. (1986), 'The internal dissemination and impact of in-house research in social services departments', *Research, Policy and Planning*, 4, 1 & 2, pp. 19–24.

Barritt, A. (1987), 'Response to "performance indicators: an alternative approach" ', unpublished.

Bennett, P. (1982), 'Female drinking and social work', in P. Bennett and S. Lupton, *Social Work and Alcohol Dependence* (Norwich: University of East Anglia).

Bhat, A. *et al.* (1988), *Britain's Black Population: A New Perspective* (Aldershot: Gower).

Booth, H. (1988), 'Identifying ethnic origin: the past, present and future of official data production', in Bhat *et al.* 1988, pp. 237–67.

Booth, T. (1986), 'Social research and policy relevance', *Research, Policy and Planning* 4, 1 & 2, pp. 15–18.

Cameron, D. and Frazer, E. (1987), *The Lust to Kill* (Cambridge: Polity Press).

Cheetham, J. *et al.* (ed.) (1981), *Social and Community Work in a Multi-Racial Society* (London: Harper and Row).

Commission for Racial Equality (1980), *1981 Census: Why the Ethnic Question is Vital* (London: CRE).

Commission for Racial Equality (1983), *CRE's submission to the House of Commons Social Services Select Committee Inquiry into Children in Care* (London: CRE).

Cooper, C. and Davidson, M. (1982), *High Pressure – Working Lives of Women Managers* (London: Fontana).

Davies, H. (1988), 'From pest control to art galleries', *Insight* 3, 49, pp. 14–15.

DHSS (1984), *Inpatient Statistics for the Mental Health Enquiry for England 1981* (London: HMSO).

Eichler, M. (1988), *Nonsexist Research Methods. A Practical Guide* (London: Allen & Unwin).

Eley, R. (1987), 'Women at the top', *Insight* 2, 12, pp. 12–14.

Etherington, S. (1989a), 'Filling the gaps', *Insight* 4, 20, pp. 20–1.

Etherington, S. (1989b), 'From the front line', *Insight* 4, 24, p. 7.

Fee, E. (1983), 'Women's nature and scientific objectivity', in M. Lowe and R. Hubbard (eds), *Women's Nature: Rationalizations of Inequality* (New York: Pergamon Press).
Fletcher, J. (1988), 'The fourth resource', *Insight* 3, 45, pp. 15–17.
Foster, J. (1987), 'Women on the wane', *Insight* 2, 50, pp. 14–15.
Foster, J. (1988a), 'On the hop', *Insight* 3, 21, pp. 20–1.
Foster, J. (1988b), 'Girls on top', *Insight* 3, 22, pp. 12–13.
Fox-Keller, E. (1985), *Reflections on Science and Gender* (New Haven: Yale University Press).

Goldberg, E. M. (1974), 'Dilemmas in social work', *Journal of Psychosomatic Research* 18.
Gostick, C. (1989), 'A good start is not enough', *Insight* 14, 8, pp. 15–16.
Gt. Britain, Parliament [1981/2] House of Commons, Social Services Committee, *1982 White Paper: Public Expenditure in the Social Services* Report 308–1.

Hadley, R. (1986), 'Beyond bureaucracy and managerialism', *Social Work Today* 18, 17, pp. 1–3.
Hale, J. (1983), 'Feminism and social work practice', in B. Jordan and N. Parton (eds), *The Political Dimensions of Social Work* (Oxford: Blackwell) pp. 167–87.
Hardingham, S. (1986), 'Angles and options', *Insight* 1, 31, pp. 12–13.
Harrison, G. *et al.* (1984), 'Psychiatric hospitalisation in Bristol II: social and clinical aspects of compusory admission', *British Journal of Psychiatry* 145, pp. 605–11.
Heginbotham, C. (1989), 'Defining the indefinable', *Insight* 14, 16, p. 21.
HMSO (1989), *Caring for People* Cmnd 849 (London: HMSO).
Hudson, A. (1988), 'Boys will be boys: masculinism and the juvenile justice system', *Critical Social Policy* 21, Spring, pp. 30–48.
Hughes, R. and Bhaduri, R. (1990), 'A model for change', *Insight* 5, 2, pp. 17, 18.
Hunt, A. (1970), 'The home help service in England and Wales', *Government Social Survey* (London: HMSO).

James, A. (1987), 'Performance and the planning process', *Insight* 2, 10, pp. 12–14.
Jones, C. (1983), *State Social Work and the Working Class* (London: Macmillan).

Kelly, A. (1989), 'The new managerialism and the welfare state', unpublished paper, Polytechnic of East London.
Knapp, M. (1987), 'Wrong numbers', *Insight* 2, 29, pp. 20–3.

Lindblom, C. (1959), 'The science of muddling through', *Public Administration Review* 19, pp. 79–88.
Lupton, C. (1985), *Moving Out. Older Teenagers Leaving Care*, Portsmouth

Social Services Research and Information Unit, Report No. 12 (Portsmouth Polytechnic).

Miller, N. (1986), 'Management information and performance measurement in the personal social services', *Social Services Research* 4/5, pp. 7–32.

Montgomery, S. (1988), 'Coming to grips with the benefits of the new technology', *Insight* 3, 19, pp. 22–4.

Nicolaus, M. (1972), 'Sociology liberation movement', in T. Pateman (ed.), *Counter Course* (Harmondsworth: Penguin) pp. 38–42.

Ohri, S. (1988), 'The politics of racism, statistics and equal opportunity: towards a black perspective', in Bhat *et al.* 1988, pp. 9–28.

Pearson, R. (1989), 'Room at the top?', *Insight* 4, 7, pp. 12–14.

Pollitt, C. (1986), 'A poor performance', *New Society*, October 3, pp. 20–1.

Popplestone, R. (1980), 'Top jobs for women: are the cards stacked against them?', *Social Work Today* 12, 4, pp. 12–15.

Roys, P. (1988), 'Social services', in Bhat *et al.* 1988, pp. 208–37.

Trow, M. (1984), 'Researchers, policy analysts and policy intellectuals', in T. Husen and M. Kogan (eds), *Educational Research and Policy: How Do They Relate?* (Oxford: Pergamon Press).

Walker, H. (1987), 'Burn out or cop out?', *Insight* 2, 41, pp. 11–13.

Warburton, W. (1989a), 'Giving a clearer indication of the KI package', *Insight*, April 11, pp. 15–17.

Warburton, W. (1989b), 'Outlying principles', *Insight* 4, 21, pp. 22–3.

Warburton, W. (1989c), 'Indicate precisely what you mean to say', *Insight* 4, 8, pp. 12–14.

Weiss, C. H. and Bucuvalas, M. J. (1980), 'Truth tests and utility tests: decision makers' frames of reference for social science research', *American Sociological Review* 45, pp. 302–13.

Wistow, G. (1987), 'Tying down the private sector', *Insight* 2, 22, pp. 14–16.

6 *Malestream training? Women, feminism and social work education*

Pam Carter, Angela Everitt and Annie Hudson

Introduction

Critical analysis of the impact of gender on social work education is still at an early stage. This is not, however, because of a lack of feminist debate. The emergence of a number of formal and semi-formal networks over the last few years has ensured much discussion (see for example Women and Social Work Education 1987). A national Women and Social Work Education conference at Ruskin College in 1986 generated a number of local networks, several of which continue to provide lively forums for discussion and action. Another conference on the subject of women and social work, held also at Ruskin College in 1989, revealed the continuing vitality of these debates. The aim of this chapter is to make such debates more public and to contribute further to feminist analysis of social work education (Smith 1986; McLeod 1987).

In writing this chapter we have drawn extensively on our own experiences as social work educators. Feminist scholarship has emphasized the importance of grounding theory in experience (Bowles and Duelli Klein 1983; Stanley and Wise 1983). Experience is not a second-rate form of knowledge: the examination of personal experience can be a crucial step in developing theoretical and empirical material. Indeed, it is only through 'understanding and analysing everyday life, where oppression as well as everything else is grounded' (Stanley and Wise 1983: 135) that we can begin to make any conceptual sense of what is going on in the world. As Du Bois has argued, a return to passionate scholarship is a prerequisite for illuminating the social world. Being passionate and explicitly partial should not be equated with 'mushiness or a focus on our own navels' (Du Bois 1983: 113).

Our use of the first-person plural – we – does not mean that our experiences have been the same: we have different social biographies and identities. We have been working in different institutions, in different parts of the country and with different groups of students. The grounding of analysis in personal experiences has both strengths and limitations; it illuminates some things and hides others. Our commonality as white middle-class women teaching on social work courses in the higher education sector means that we have many privileges and considerable power. Our experiences are thereby inevitably limited; we therefore acknowledge fully that it is impossible and even dangerous always to generalize from our own experiences. Racism, heterosexism and classism are just as much determining influences as sexism on social work education. In what follows then, we have endeavoured to explore how oppressions other than gender connect with social work education's institutionalized sexism.

Our experience has been largely gained through teaching on courses awarding the Certificate of Qualification in Social Work (CQSW); we have had little involvement in those courses which award the Certificate in Social Service (CSS). However, we hope that many of the themes addressed here transcend different sectors of social work education, and that women involved in CSS will find common features. Our focus on education and training for social work, rather than that for other social services personnel such as home care organizers or care assistants, further defines the scope of the discussion.

Because social work education is currently undergoing considerable change, the articulation of feminist perspectives is particularly urgent. In the course of the 1990s the CQSW and CSS are to be replaced by the new Diploma in Social Work (DipSW) (CCETSW 1989a). There will continue to be different routes to the DipSW (college-based and employment-based), and there should be more flexibility in provision through modular, distance learning and part-time programmes. The new diploma reveals the determination by CCETSW to impose standardized national criteria for the social work qualification in place of the old system, which allows for considerable local discretion and interpretation. Students will thus be expected to demonstrate that they have achieved a minimum level of competence in relation to specified knowledge, skills and values for social work practice (CCETSW, 1989b).

The responsibility of college-based educators for CQSW social work courses is to give way to partnership with social work agencies. CCETSW will 'only consider for approval DipSW programmes submitted jointly by educational institutions and social service agencies' (CCETSW 1989b: 22). Such programme providers are responsible not only for overseeing the admissions and assessment policies, but also for ensuring that the 'outcomes' as specified in the statement of requirements are achieved, and that the resources required are secured. Finally, CCETSW's anti-discriminatory strategy requires that students qualifying with the DipSW should be prepared for 'ethnically sensitive practice'. They should be able to 'challenge and confront institutional and other forms of racism' and 'other forms of discrimination' (CCETSW 1989b: 10).

Though it is difficult to predict how CCETSW's anti-discriminatory policies will unfold, many of their underlying principles are very welcome. For example, the fact that DipSW students will have to undergo training and assessment in anti-discriminatory practice is an important step forward. It is vital that the freedom of educators to be critical is maintained to ensure that such requirements are not merely tokenistic. Effective collaboration between educators in both colleges and the field requires a commitment to broader educational goals as well as to narrow vocational objectives. One area of concern is the potential drift towards increasing agency management control of social work education (Jones 1989; Parsloe 1990). This drift is not encouraging for feminist scholarship and practice in social work, for women involved in social work education, or for anti-discriminatory education and practice.

The planned transformation of social work education will also affect training for women in the social care sector (for example, home care assistants, childminders and residential care assistants). Indeed the new Certificate in Social Care is designed to encourage the expansion of education in these hitherto neglected areas, in which the majority of staff are women and many are black (Phillipson 1988). CCETSW presents the new Certificate in Social Care as a major step forward in opening up social services training and education.

> [It] will cater for the access needs of disadvantaged groups, such as ethnic minorities, women joining or rejoining the labour market and people changing careers, as well as the in-service training needs of staff (CCETSW 1987: 27).

However, the consolidation of the Certificate in Social Care qualification will also have the effect of reinforcing the distinction between professionally qualified social workers and vocationally trained social care workers. On the one hand CCETSW claims to be espousing equal opportunities, but on the other it helps to maintain divisions in the workforce on gender and racial lines.

Our discussion is organized around three themes; first, we consider the position of women as students, then as staff. The final section reflects on the impact of feminism on the social work education curriculum.

Women social work students: training for change or control?

Education in British society has a major role in reproducing and sometimes restructuring the labour force (Bowles and Gintis 1976; Education Group CCCS 1981). Social work education helps to create employment patterns in which women, black and working-class people are disproportionately concentrated in lower status and less well paid jobs. Meanwhile white middle-class men claim power and prestige in the higher echelons of social work (Howe 1986; Dominelli 1988; Hanmer and Statham 1988; also Lupton in this volume). What are the mechanisms and values within social work education that contribute to such a divided workforce?

Institutions of higher education have been responsible for the selection and licensing of social workers. Social work education has provided access to higher education and a professional career for a substantial number of working-class, black, mature and women students. However, the proportions of black and working-class people who become social work students do not begin to approximate to the need for these groups to be represented in the social work workforce (Community Care 1987). Such patterns reveal a hidden function of social work education: that of restricting and controlling access to the profession.

To make sense of the connections between social work education and employment patterns we analyse data concerning student intakes to different types of social work education and training. Table 6.1 shows how women's position in social work education changed between 1980 and 1987.

On first inspection the table suggests not only that women have fared equitably in terms of selection to social work courses, but also that during the 1980s their relative position improved. Women predominate in every form of training route and every type of course. Closer reading of these patterns reveals, however, that their relative concentration on courses varies considerably. In 1987 women were particularly highly represented in four-year undergraduate courses, three-year courses and on pre-qualification courses (ICSC and PCSC). By contrast women constituted only 55 per cent of the total entry on to post-qualifying courses. In terms of CQSW courses, the highest proportion of male entrants is in two-year post-graduate CQSW courses (34 per cent of total in 1987). Such courses often offer a master's (*sic*) degree – an award which may prove an asset in subsequent career terms. More detailed gendered breakdowns of intakes to different types of post-qualifying courses would be revealing, as indeed would figures for the intakes to other non-CCETSW approved post-qualifying courses, and particularly to management training courses.

Table 6.1 Women's position in social work education 1980–7

Student intake by sex (%) 1980 and 1987 all CCETSW-Approved Courses, United Kingdom

	Female 1980	(%) 1987	Male 1980	(%) 1987	Total 1980	1987
Certificate of qualification in Social Work (CQSW)						
1 year post-graduate	69	72	31	28	793	581
2 year post-graduate	62	66	38	34	682	673
4 year undergraduate	73	80	27	20	323	397
2 year non-graduate	61	72	39	28	1894	1533
3 year (extended courses)	85	93	15	7	98	119
Total CQSW	65	77	35	23	3790	3303
Certificate in Social Service (CSS)	69	69	31	31	1076	1642
Post-qualifying studies (PQS)	50	55	51	45	210	249
In-service Certificate in Social Care (ICSC)	78	80	22	20	3347	4533
Preliminary Certificate in Social Care (PCSC)	93	89	7	11	2261	2223

Sources: CCETSW 1981: 8; 1988b: 8. (Figures have been rounded up for comparison.)

It may seem surprising that CSS schemes, which cater primarily for those workers (predominantly women) in residential and day care, recruit proportionately fewer women than three out of the five CQSW routes. Though the residential and day care sector has traditionally been regarded as an area of female employment, the proportion of men in management grades in this sector is markedly greater than in basic care assistant grades (Howe 1986). The above figures suggest that CSS training has reinforced this differential. Now that the DipSW has removed the difference (and the implicit status differential) between CQSW and CSS, we may find that professional qualifying training opportunities for women and other socially disadvantaged groups (particularly for those with minimal formal educational qualifications) will be restricted. Instead, such groups will be increasingly directed to the shorter and less marketable pre-qualification ICSC and PCSC courses.

Numerical data, however, provide only a limited guide to power relations in social work education. What can we learn from the ways in which the experiences of women as social work students are structured? Returning to study is always a challenge for mature students, but for black women and working-class women there are particular obstacles to negotiate. The Taking Liberties Collective (which includes women who have been on CQSW courses) have presented an eloquent account of the ways in which working-class and black women have to 'move heaven and earth' to make their studies possible;

> Keeping the home fires burning, looking after children, doing domestic work and dealing with the opposition, act as the preliminary heats designed to weed out all but the most dedicated (Taking Liberties Collective 1989: 73).

From start to finish such women have to wage battles against their own and others' expectations about their capacity to negotiate successfully the educational system (essay writing, talking in seminars, presenting a 'professional' image on placements and so on). Only 'grim determination' (Taking Liberties Collective 1989: 88) enables such women to survive the obstacle courses of social work training. Cuts in higher education and increasing employer control stack the dice even more heavily against black and working-class women.

The centrality of the care and control discourse in contemporary state social work is now widely recognized (Day 1981; Rojek, Peacock and Collins 1988). Feminist research and action has shown how repairing or caring, and regulating or controlling, are highly gendered, and that the links between the two are often disguised (Dale and Foster 1986; Hanmer and Statham 1988). Caring both links and divides female professionals and female clients. Women as social work professionals police and control the caring abilities of clients. 'Control' in these relationships is often presented as care and concern. No wonder then that the question of women social workers assuming care and control roles is a confusing area for feminist social workers (Wise 1985). It is not so widely recognized that similar processes operate inside social work education; of particular concern is how social work education can most appropriately challenge the control of women through expectations of various kinds of caring behaviour, leaving men to manage and control. Social work education can either reproduce or challenge such expectations for women students in their personal and professional lives.

The language of care and control has played a major role in structuring the gendered relations of social work education. Entry to a social work training course involves socialization into values which are congruent with both repairing and regulating roles. An adaptation of Bernstein's notions of visible and invisible pedagogies (Bernstein 1977), suggests that social work education relies more heavily on the latter than the former. Hierarchical relationships between staff and students and the criteria for licensing are implicit rather than explicit in the rules and principles of social work education. The student–tutor/practice teacher relationship is often formally presented as a means of encouraging professional development (care), but in reality the relationship is greatly influenced by the tutor's or practice teacher's authority and power to assess the student. This modelling of the confused nature of care and control, exercised through 'friendly' relationships, needs to be made more visible.

The lack of social distance between tutor or practice teacher and student compared with that between social worker and client compounds the confusion about care and control. The relationship can more easily be interpreted as one between colleagues or friends rather than between educators and students. Where this involves male tutors monitoring female students, the latter can be placed in particularly vulnerable positions. Instances of sexual harassment in social work are rarely 'extreme and terrible, but small, mundane and accumulating' (Wise and Stanley 1987: 98). Naming such instances is not easy, particularly when the hierarchy between male teacher and female student is invisible. When, for example, does a male hug in an experiential groupwork session become an intrusion; and if the woman feels reluctant to so 'engage' does she become defined as 'over-defended' and 'unfeeling'?

Ignoring the role of tutors and practice teachers as assessors may in reality mean discriminating against female, black and other socially disadvantaged students. The lack of explicit and shared expectations of students, and the lack of accountability of assessors for many of their decisions (particularly in relation to practice assessment) inhibits equity and justice (Borland *et al.* 1988). When it comes to making pass/fail decisions, assessors may rely on their subjective evaluations. Those who conform more neatly with assessors' unstated notions of what makes for a 'good' social worker are clearly better placed than those who are less conforming. Lesbian or gay students, for example, whose lifestyles and politics may be regarded as 'unacceptable' by a particular tutor or practice teacher, may as a result be judged to be 'unacceptable' for social work practice. In contrast, students who have failed to develop a coherent anti-racist and anti-sexist practice can slip by on the nod.

A sharper focus on the educational task and the explicit development of appropriate educational relationships should encourage students and staff alike to be more critical and explicit about what constitutes an effective practitioner.

'The boys' game'? Women as social work educators

Women assume the role of social work educator in a variety of contexts (as practice teachers, student unit organizers, training officers and college-based teachers) and in a wide range of institutions (higher education, further education, student units and social work agencies). While we concentrate here on the college sector, it is striking that in all these areas similar patterns of vertical and horizontal segregation can be found.

First, it is clear that men predominate in higher education. In the 1989 Association of University Teachers' survey, for example, in the group which includes social sciences (and thus usually social work), 78.7 per cent of teaching and research staff were male, compared with 93.3 per cent in engineering and technologies (Association of University Teachers 1989). At one of our institutions, a large polytechnic, 100 per cent of the directorate and deans are men, 90 per cent of the heads of departments are men, as are 91 per cent of principal lecturers, 76 per cent of senior lecturers and 60 per cent of lecturers. By contrast, among the students in the same institution women are in the majority in all but the pure and applied sciences.

Second, women are most likely to be found in the humanities and social science sectors, as opposed to the 'purer' and more established disciplines such as science, law and engineering. Such patterns reflect gender divisions which prescribe that women should concentrate on 'softer' academic studies such as social work and the arts. Within social work, lecturers are more likely than basic grade social workers to be male. Hence practice teachers are more likely than college lecturers to be women. Women involved in social work teaching and research occupy relatively low status positions. The absence of black women in social work education is, predictably, even more marked. Though there is currently no official data, a cursory acquaintance with the staff groups of the majority of social work courses highlights how black women in social work education are noticeable by their absence. Notwithstanding a couple of 'notable exception' courses, the contribution of black women to social work education and research has, by and large, remained unacknowledged and invisible.

Similar processes to those that have blocked the appointment of women into social work management also operate in social work education. As social work's professional 'respectability' has been enhanced, so the prestige of social work education has made it more attractive to men. Indeed status often compensates for money: a professor's salary, for example, compares unfavourably with that of a social services director or chief probation officer.

Men are widely regarded as being more suitable than women for the academic tasks of 'theorizing' and undertaking research. Indeed canons of academic 'wisdom' place considerable emphasis on the capacity of would-be recruits to be analytic, rational and intellectually confident. Such qualities are clearly relevant; the problem is that only 'exceptional' women are seen as having such attributes. As a result women often find it difficult to envisage themselves as competent in such spheres. The schooling of female social workers to assume that their capacities are best deployed in face-to-face work rather than in management or in academia, together with covert discrimination by academic institutions, has restricted women's presence in more senior academic levels of social work education.

Our socialization as women is a further constraint on us developing confidence in the 'arcane' and 'rather forbidding' worlds of theory and academia:

> And, particularly if we are women, we will have been encouraged to think of 'theory' as special, not a part of everyday life; something produced by clever people (who just happen to be men), not by us (Stanley and Wise 1983: 33).

It is no wonder that many black and white women lack the necessary self-assurance to make a contribution to social work's research base.

By contrast, men are more likely to consider themselves appropriate candidates for senior academic positions. Appointments committees, concerned to demonstrate academic credibility, look favourably on a curriculum vitae that includes a long list of publications and suggests the ability to haul in large research grants. We need to question not only who has the time for writing and research, but also who decides, and upon what criteria, what is published and what is funded.

The slow and uneven implementation of equal opportunities policies in higher education has delayed the appointment of women to senior positions. Furthermore, it is important to reflect critically on the patterns of appointment to more senior positions: who is appointed, and on whose terms? (Everitt 1990). The criteria are rarely made explicit, and decisions are not systematically monitored for different forms of discriminatory bias. Additionally, because appointment committees tend to be dominated by more senior staff, they are generally composed of a majority of white, middle-class men.

Other factors have also constrained the power and influence of women in academic posts. While part-time lectureships may be more attractive for women with children or other dependants, in many institutions such lecturers are often on temporary or short-term contracts. This means that part-time staff cannot apply for promotion, nor do they have automatic membership of decision-making bodies such as departmental and faculty boards. Indeed, at least one educational institution that we know of has explicitly stated that 'part-time staff tend not to be given the same level of responsibilities . . . as full-time staff, *because of the intermittent nature of their commitment, and that the Department's expectations of part-time staff tend to be lower*' (our emphasis).[1] With such policies, it is no wonder that many women educators have so much difficulty in gaining promotion.

The *perceived* ability of candidates to undertake research and to command research funds is now at a premium; consequently, the ability to establish appropriate and effective relationships with students and to teach competently is deemed of less importance. By virtue of their more senior positions, men are often better placed to be entrepreneurs and to go out and 'hunt' for research and consultancy activities. Meanwhile, back at the ranch, their female counterparts are expected to 'keep the homes fires burning' through teaching and tutoring activities.

Abramowitz' study of social work education in Israel suggests that, in that country at least, women take on a disproportionate responsibility for class work (Abramowitz 1985). Although similar evidence is not available for Britain, these findings certainly echo our experience. The ideologies of femininity and caring affect women as social work educators as well as students. It is our experience that women staff who do not give all their time to their students, and engage in writing and research, are regarded as 'uncaring'. Women staff are also expected to provide women students with the support that they fail to get from sexist male staff. Should we, as women staff, take on extra work with women students?

The structure of many women's lives does not fit in well with performing academic tasks. Women with children or other dependants find it particularly difficult to get long periods without interruption for writing and research, while men who are 'serviced' domestically by female partners are at a significant advantage. Women frequently find it practically impossible to get away to conferences and other professional gatherings. In any case, for many women, much ambivalence surrounds such events given the male, heterosexual culture that frequently prevails.

CCETSW's concern to institutionalize a more collaborative approach to social work training may prove to be an additional force in consolidating white male decision-making power. It is too early to provide substantive evidence of such trends, but it is our experience that there are good grounds for such fears. The greater likelihood of white middle-class men being in senior decision-making positions in both agencies and colleges fuels concerns about plans for collaboration and partnership. Many agencies have regarded CSS as the apotheosis of social work education, particularly with regard to collaboration and partnership; if partnership models lay emphasis on employer control, then programme provider arrangements will exacerbate rather than increase the relative powerlessness of women social work educators in both colleges and agencies.

Feminism and its challenges to the curriculum

The social work education curriculum is an obvious and crucial site for ensuring that the complexity of gender-related issues is appropriately addressed in social work training and education. Unfortunately, feminist perspectives and experiences have frequently been regarded at best as irrelevant, and at worst as actively damaging to the enterprise of equipping students for the hurly-burly of social work practice. A number of aspects of the curriculum warrant attention: these include consideration of the role of women and the status of feminism in defining social work's theoretical base; and the content and methods for addressing feminist issues within social work courses.

Feminists working within and outside the social sciences have rigorously analysed the construction of knowledge and have questioned the extent that its theories address the realities of women's experiences. Appeals for so-called 'objectivity' particularly have had to be challenged to reveal their underlying biases and values (Stanley and Wise 1983; see also Lupton in this volume). Traditional definitions of 'acceptable' social science theory have been influential in shaping much of social work's institutionalized discrimination against, for example, black people, women, lesbians and gay men and old people. Within social work, feminist practitioners and writers have highlighted how 'commonsense' assumptions about 'good practice' must constantly be scrutinized for their (sometimes unwitting) assumptions about women's needs and roles (Hanmer and Statham 1988; Dominelli and McLeod 1989; Hudson 1989).

Feminists have also examined research methods, raising major questions about the validity, accountability and power relations within much research (Roberts 1981; Stanley and Wise 1983). Feminist research methodology, developed from this critique, can make a significant contribution to social work in that 'it generates its problematics from the perspective of women's experiences' (Harding 1987: 7).

The equation of theory with 'men's work' has given men in

social work disproportionate control of the process of creating knowledge. As Wise has pointed out:

> Put simply, while women remain as the practitioners whose time is occupied in doing the work, male academics will have greater space and time to describe and theorise about it (Wise 1988: xiv).

Data from the United States illustrates how, in America at least, women have been less involved in social work research and writing than their male counterparts (Kirk and Rosenblatt 1984). These patterns suggest that women's voice in the process of theorizing about social work practice is considerably less than it should be. So, while women have created the 'meanings' in the world of practice, in academic social work men have appropriated this role (Davis 1985).

Women social workers, through their numerically dominant role as front-line workers, are the producers of knowledge, while men, because of their relative dominance in academia, enjoy relatively greater power in defining 'legitimate' social work theory. Women's contributions to social work theory are thereby frequently rendered invisible. It may not be an exaggeration to suggest that somewhere along the line there has been a 'rip off' of women's ideas and experiences.

Feminist scholarship and research has much to offer to the social work curriculum. The prejudicial myths and negative stereotypes of feminist students and staff are, however, as widespread within social work education as they are in social work agencies. Asserting the central importance of gender and women's issues in the curriculum is often regarded as 'unfeminine' and 'aggressive'. We have had many experiences of situations in which support of feminist endeavours has been much more forthcoming from students than from staff. Despite being formally conversant with the language of anti-sexist discourse, many male (and some female) educators have failed to internalize its importance as an everyday dimension of educational and social work practice. Feminism seems to touch a raw nerve in the personal and professional identity of many male educators. When challenges are made to the 'here and now' practice of a particular institution or staff group, traditional prejudices often surface. The 'in this staff group, men are innocent till proven guilty' response to these 'awkward' women asserting their collective voice suggests that feminism is often perceived as a castrating force.

The coherent integration of knowledge about, and skills for addressing, different sources of oppression, is fundamental to effective learning methods. Yet on many courses teaching about gender, race, class, sexual identity and age is compartmentalized as if each is assumed to be totally separate from the other, rather than all being interconnected facets of people's lives. If white women educators and students are to take seriously black women's critique of white feminism (Bryan, Dadzie and Scafe 1985; Ahmed 1986) then the separation of teaching about gender from other forms of social inequality is highly problematic.

When issues such as anti-racism or anti-sexism are separated from the 'mainstream' curriculum, students and staff are discouraged from implementing the complexities of anti-discriminatory principles into everyday practice. Teaching about gender, race, class, age, able-bodiedness and sexuality is inevitably a difficult and challenging task. It is impossible to contain such issues within formal subject boundaries and the 'classroom walls'. Feminist social work, like anti-racist practice, will never be a comfortable component of the curriculum. Jane Thompson has commented on the tendency of 'women's studies' to produce 'resistance' within institutions:

> They offer not merely a discrete view of the world within the confines of a 'new subject specialism', but a commentary on the rest of the curriculum and of academia (Thompson 1983: 112).

In our experience, teaching gender on social work courses can evolve into a critique of other parts of the course. For example, what happens when, through considering the impact of gender, women tutees begin to challenge their male tutors? What happens when women staff make it legitimate to reject heterosexual relationships? Or what happens when black students in practice placements challenge the racism of social work agencies? Feminism is inevitably subversive. No wonder then that feminists are often seen as 'troublemakers'. Specific groups of women are particularly vulnerable: women lecturers and students who are black, working-class and/or lesbian are particularly likely to be the focus of such attacks.

The exploration of the impact of social inequalities may indeed appear to be divisive of both staff and student groups. For example, female students may voice anger and resentment at the way in which male students and staff 'posture' about anti-sexism but are, in reality, reluctant to accept personal responsibility for everyday manifestations of sexism. Yet learning about gender can be as creative and productive as it is potentially uncomfortable. For many students, male as well as female, it can become a major learning platform. It often results in excellent written work, dissertations, research projects, creative initiatives on placements, and may even lead to the recasting of identities and self-assumptions.

More than half of students' experiences of social work education takes place in practice agencies. Despite images of rampant vocationalism, many practice teachers, practitioners and some training officers are deeply committed to critical and analytic approaches to practice and to the generation of knowledge for social work. It is often they who push the educational institutions into looking more critically at the curriculum, particularly in relation to anti-sexism and anti-racism. Low staff turnover and lack of involvement in practice and research in many academic departments have meant that many educators have been slow to develop strong anti-racist and anti-sexist perspectives. In contrast, some practice teachers and agencies have been very prominent in raising these issues and in making sure that courses keep them on the agenda. In the past few years a number of practice teachers have pioneered feminist and anti-racist social work and community work. Such agencies provide a crucial knowledge base and resource for feminists in social work education.

However, in many agencies anti-discriminatory practice is barely on the agenda. While practice placements in these agencies offer important opportunities in learning to devise strategies for change, the experience of doing so can be very demanding and stressful. CCETSW's policies for accrediting both individual practice teachers and agencies for practice teaching purport to tackle these issues (CCETSW 1988b). Its proposals, however, seem naive in relation to the scale of the change needed and the depth of resistance that is likely to be encountered. As yet CCETSW has not evolved coherent strategies for enabling educators both in colleges and in agencies to persuade reluctant agencies to go beyond, or even as far as, bland anti-discriminatory statements.

Finally, there are grounds for considerable disquiet about the marginal role allocated by CCETSW to the social science disciplines in its proposals for the DipSW:

> 'For the award of the DSW, academic disciplines should only be assessed with relevance to social work practice' (CCETSW 1989a: 5).

This tendency to dichotomize social work and social science theory is potentially damaging to the development of critical practice. It underlines the need to sustain and increase the impact of feminism and other anti-discriminatory perspectives. Social work and social work education have much to gain from the feminist commitment to develop theory and practice alongside each other. Take, for example, the issue of domestic violence; the Women's Aid movement has not only directly confronted traditional ideas about 'why' some women are battered, but it has also demonstrated alternative and practical ways of responding to women at the receiving end of such violence (Pahl 1985; Dobash and Dobash 1987).

The development of feminist theory and practice in social work education is nonetheless also equally dependent on feminists themselves being open and alert to the complexities of women's experiences. If our own ideas and practices are not subjected to constant evaluation and critique, then we risk establishing yet another set of orthodoxies.

As social work educators we identify feminism with critical education and analysis, rather than with the development of technical skills and competencies. Social workers must obviously be skilled and competent but this can only arise out of a set of values that is critical of the subtle impacts of social work's dominant ideologies. Social work education has a key role to play in enhancing the critical debates and analysis that are so crucial to anti-discriminatory practice. Whether 'partnerships' between colleges and agencies can retain a commitment to education and critical debate, as opposed to crude vocationalism, must be the key question for social work education in the 1990s.

Note

1 Personal communication.

References

Abramowitz, N. (1985), 'Status of women on faculty and status of women's studies Israeli Schools of Social Work', *Social Work Education* 4, 3, pp. 3–6.

Ahmed, S. (1986), 'Cultural racism in work with Asian women and girls', in Ahmed, S., Cheetham, J. and Small, J. (eds), *Social Work with Black Children and their Families* (London: Batsford) pp. 140–54.

Association of University Teachers (1989), *Distribution of Women in the Academic and Related Workforce in UK Universities* (London: Association of University Teachers).

Bernstein, B. (1977), *Class, Codes and Control, Volume 3: Towards a Theory of Educational Transmissions* (London: Routledge and Kegan Paul).

Borland, M., Hudson, A., Hughes, B. and Worrall, A. (1988), 'An approach to the management of the assessment of practice placements', *British Journal of Social Work* 18, 3, pp. 269–87.

Bowles, G. and Duelli Klein, R. (1983), 'Introduction: theories of Women's Studies and the autonomy/integration debate', in G. Bowles and R. Duelli Klein (eds), *Theories of Women's Studies* (London: Routledge and Kegan Paul) pp. 1–26.

Bowles, S. and Gintis, H. (1976), *Schooling in Capitalist America* (London: Routledge and Kegan Paul).

Bryan, B., Dadzie, S. and Scafe, S. (1985), *The Heart of the Race: Black Women's Lives in Britain* (London: Virago).

CCETSW (1981), *Annual Returns by Courses* (London: CCETSW).
CCETSW (1987), *Care for Tomorrow* (London: CCETSW).
CCETSW (1988a), *Annual Returns by Courses* (London: CCETSW).
CCETSW (1988b), *Accreditation of Agencies and Practice Teachers in Social Work Education* Paper 26:2 (London: CCETSW).
CCETSW (1989a), *Proposal for a Diploma in Social Work (DSW)* (London: CCETSW).
CCETSW (1989b), *Regulations for Programmes Leading to the Diploma in Social Work* (London: CCETSW).
Community Care (1987), 'Inside: anti-racist education for social workers', *Community Care*, October 29, pp. i–viii.

Dale, P. and Foster, P. (1986), *Feminists and State Welfare* (London: Routledge and Kegan Paul).
Davis, L. V. (1985), 'Female and male voices in social work', *Social Work* 30, 2, pp. 106–13.
Day, P. (1981), *Social Work and Social Control* (London: Tavistock).
Dobash, R. E. and Dobash, R. P. (1987), 'The response of the British and American women's movements to violence against women', in J. Hanmer and M. Maynard (eds) (1987), *Women, Violence and Social Control* (Basingstoke: Macmillan) pp. 169–79.
Dominelli, L. (1988), *Anti-Racist Social Work* (Basingstoke: Macmillan).
Dominelli, L. and McLeod, E. (1989), *Feminist Social Work* (Basingstoke: Macmillan).
Du Bois, B. (1983), 'Passionate scholarship: notes on values, knowledge and method in feminist social science', in Bowles and Duelli Klein 1983, pp. 105–16.

Education Group, Centre for Contemporary Cultural Studies (CCCS) (1981), *Unpopular Education: Schooling and Social Democracy in England since 1914* (London: Hutchinson).
Everitt, A. (1990), 'Will women managers save social work?', in P. Carter, T. Jeffs and M. Smith (eds), *Social Work and Social Welfare Yearbook 2* (Milton Keynes: Open University Press) pp. 134–48.

Hanmer, J. and Statham, D. (1988), *Women and Social Work* (Basingstoke: Macmillan).
Harding, S. (1987), 'Is there a feminist method?', in S. Harding (ed.), *Feminism and Methodology* (Milton Keynes: Open University Press) pp. 1–14.
Howe, D. (1986), 'The segregation of women and their work in the personal social services', *Critical Social Policy* 15, pp. 21–36.
Hudson, A. (1989), 'Changing perspectives: feminism, gender and social work', in M. Langan and P. Lee (eds), *Radical Social Work Today* (London: Unwin Hyman) pp. 70–96.

Jones, C. (1989), 'The end of the road? Issues in social work education', in P. Carter, T. Jeffs and M. Smith (eds), *Social Work and Social Welfare Yearbook 1* (Milton Keynes: Open University Press) pp. 204–16.

Kirk, S. and Rosenblatt, A. (1984), 'The contribution of women faculty members to social work journals', *Social Work* 29 (1), pp. 67–9.

McLeod, E. (1987), 'Some lessons from teaching feminist social work', *Social Work Education* 7, 1, pp. 29–37.

Pahl, J. (1985), 'Refuges for battered women: ideology and action', in *Feminist Review* 19, pp. 25–43.

Parsloe, P. (1990), 'Future of social work education: recovering from "Care for Tomorrow" ', in P. Carter, T. Jeffs and M. Smith 1990, pp. 197–210.

Phillipson, J. (1988), 'The complexities of caring: developing a feminist approach to training staff in a residential setting', *Social Work Education* 7, 3, pp. 3–6.

Roberts, H. (ed.) (1981), *Doing Feminist Research* (London: Routledge and Kegan Paul).

Rojek, C., Peacock, G. and Collins, S. (1988), *Social Work and Received Ideas* (London: Routledge).

Smith, B. (1986), 'The case for women's studies in social work education', in H. Marchant and B. Wearing (eds), *Gender Reclaimed: Women in Social Work* (Sydney: Hale and Iremonger) pp. 201–11.

Stanley, L. and Wise, S. (1983), *Breaking Out: Feminist Consciousness and Feminist Research* (London: Routledge and Kegan Paul).

Taking Liberties Collective (1989), *Learning the Hard Way: Women's Oppression in Men's Education* (Basingstoke: Macmillan).

Thompson, J. (1983), *Learning Liberation: Women's Response to Men's Education* (Beckenham: Croom Helm).

Wise, S. (1985), 'Becoming a feminist social worker', *Studies in Sexual Politics* 6 (Manchester: Department of Sociology, University of Manchester).

Wise, S. (1988), 'Doing feminist social work: an annotated bibliography and introductory essay', *Studies in Sexual Politics* 21 (Manchester: Department of Sociology, University of Manchester).

Wise, S. and Stanley, L. (1987), *Georgie Porgie: Sexual Harassment in Everyday Life* (London: Pandora Press).

Women and Social Work Education (1987), *Women and Social Work Education: Study Conference Report of the Conference Planning Group* (Manchester: Department of Social Policy and Social Work, University of Manchester).

7 *The child sexual abuse 'industry' and gender relations in social work*

Annie Hudson

Introduction

In the mid-1980s child sexual abuse quite suddenly became a high-profile media 'story'. The sudden upsurge in the numbers of children taken into local authority care as a result of a 'diagnosis' of child sexual abuse provoked angry reactions from parents, certain sections of the media, and MPs, amongst others. The resulting public inquiry under Lord Justice Butler-Sloss focused attention both on the plight of children who had been sexually abused and on appropriate methods of dealing with the problem (HMSO 1988).

In Britain in the 1880s issues of 'white slavery', child prostitution and incest were the focus of considerable, if often prurient, concern, in spite of the fact that the sexual abuse of children had been a taboo for the best part of a century before. In response, feminists linked up with philanthropists and evangelicals to promote the rescue and rehabilitation of those who had been subjected to the 'horrors and abominations' of incest (Mearns 1883, quoted in Wohl 1978: 207). Looking back at the debates of the 1880s and 1980s reveals important similarities, and differences, in perceptions of the problem of child sexual abuse and how it should be tackled. I begin this chapter by looking in more detail at the earlier campaigns, and their lessons for today.

The issue of child sexual abuse did not re-emerge spontaneously in Cleveland in 1987. Its dramatic reappearance was the culmination of more than a decade in which the issue was gradually being broached by activists within the women's movement, particularly by women involved in rape crisis centres, and in other forums where women had become aware that child sexual abuse was a feature of the lives of many women. The women's movement had thereby exposed the sexual abuse of children as yet another manifestation of male supremacy and power within the family.

One of the most significant outcomes of the Cleveland crisis has been the creation of a new welfare industry around child sexual abuse issues, which largely excludes the feminist influence which had been so crucial in bringing the issue to public attention. This process, and its consequences, constitute the second theme of this chapter. As child sexual abuse has become a major sphere of public concern and medico-social intervention, so have men assumed disproportionate control and influence. This has come about through their ability to control professional debates, and through their management of agencies with responsibility for dealing with child sexual abuse. In interpreting the problem and in social interventions, medical and psychological models have replaced questions of gender relations and family structures.

Yet child sexual abuse continues to present complex challenges for social workers. While the problem is now at least acknowledged rather than being denied, the state has not made available the resources to ensure appropriate and sensitive care for children and adults. In 1989, for example, a MORI poll suggested that 78 per cent of all social services departments had insufficient resources to cope with child sexual abuse work (Morris 1989). Child sexual abuse poses, in the sharpest form, the tension between being counsellor and befriender or enforcer of statutory powers (Satyamurti 1979; Jones 1983). The third theme of this chapter is to consider how feminist social workers can establish forms of practice which ensure appropriate protection for children, without undermining their rights or those of their parents.

'What to do about child sexual abuse?': comparing the 1880s and the 1990s

During the late 1880s the sexual abuse of children was one of a number of issues of public morality and private rights around which major debates and campaigns took place (Weeks 1981; Jeffreys 1985). An uneasy alliance between campaigners for 'social purity', feminists, radical philanthropists, church-people, and politicians, challenged the secrecy and denial that had previously surrounded discussions of 'incest'.

The ideologies and interests of groups within this alliance were by no means identical or complementary. The feminist commitment to publicizing the scale of child sexual abuse arose from a concern to expose the double standard which demanded the purity of woman at the same time as condoning the systematic exploitation of girls and young women. A number of such feminists joined the National Vigilance Association (NVA) which mounted a crusade against vice and immorality (Jeffreys 1985).

Male and female social purist campaigners regarded the moral rearmament of the urban and dispossessed poor as only attainable through adherence to the gospel of family life. The association between moral crusading and child protection was reflected in the links between the NVA and the newly founded National Society for the Prevention of Cruelty to Children (NSPCC) (Bailey and Blackburn 1979). Rev. Ben Waugh, for example, was both the founding director of the NSPCC and a member of the NVA council. Both organizations were preoccupied with upholding bourgeois family values through an emphasis on moral propriety and religion. (The appointment in 1989 of Margaret Thatcher as a vice-president of the NSPCC (Community Care 1989a) reveals the continuity of a commitment to Victorian values in the sphere of child protection.)

In the 1980s, welfare professionals have assumed the role, formerly occupied by 'social purity' campaigners, of defining the parameters of public debates around child sexual abuse. Yet the interventions of right wing political forces concerned to use the issue of child sexual abuse to promote 'traditional' (conservative) family values is a common theme from the 1880s to 1990s. Valerie Riches, the secretary of Family and Youth Concern (a right wing pro-family pressure group) exemplifies this approach:

> Trying to tackle the problem of child sex abuse by allocating further resources for more services, without at the same time strengthening the traditional family, is like mopping up the bathwater while the bath is still overflowing (Riches 1990).

In both late Victorian and contemporary debate, commentators have alleged that child sexual abuse is peculiar to particular social groups or classes. In the past the notion that 'incest' was commonplace among the urban poor was a perennial theme (Wohl 1970; Jeffreys 1985; Gordon 1989). Rev. Andrew Mearns' famous pamphlet 'Bitter Cry of Outcast London', first published in 1884, argued, for example, that inadequate urban housing had caused the 'sinking' of some sections of the working class into this most sinful of sins (Wohl 1970). Most campaigners and policy-makers in the 1880s failed to make any connection between child sexual abuse and prevailing ideologies of masculinity. The 'sense of superiority' (Gordon 1989: 215) implicit in the depiction of child sexual abuse as the deviant behaviour of the demoralized poor absolved 'normal' and supposedly 'respectable' families from any taint of suspicion – prejudices which persist to this day.

Victorian society regarded sexual abuse as a grossly deviant departure from a family norm of unquestioned virtue and propriety. Hence the appropriate response was to inculcate due respect for the sanctity of family life among those who had deviated from its norms. By contrast today such ideas have been replaced by notions of pathology and treatment. No longer, moreover, are clerics seen as playing a central role in ridding society of this social blight. Instead, it is the 'psy' professionals (Donzelot 1980) who have been assigned the primary defining and expert role.

The Victorians were reluctant to use the civil law to intervene in the private sphere of the family, and delayed in making 'incest' a criminal rather than an ecclesiastic offence (Wohl 1978). The concern that an over-zealous legal approach would 'do an infinite amount of mischief' and lead to the unjust prosecution of men meant that it was not until 1908 that 'incest' was defined as a criminal offence (Bailey and Blackburn 1979). Even though the legal framework governing responses to child sexual abuse has been greatly extended, great ambivalence still remains about using the criminal law as a mechanism for dealing with child sexual abuse. The law concerning child sexual abuse is both confusing and contradictory (Woodcraft 1988; Viinikka 1989). Although severe penalties for such offences are prescribed, in practice the execution of these laws tends to place the child rather than the adult perpetrator on trial.

Such presumptions emerge again and again in criminal trials, when children are, for example, continually 'accused' of being 'seductive' and 'responsible' for the abuse (Driver 1989). The maximum punishment for the crime of incest is life imprisonment when the child is under 13 years, but only seven years if she (or he) is above this age. Sentencing guidelines issued in 1989 reiterated notions that the severity of the abuse, and the maximum punishment thereby decreed, should negatively correlate with the age of the 'victim'. This was apparent in a comment by one of the Appeal Court Judges who issued these guidelines:

> The older the girl, the greater the possibility that she may have been willing or even *the instigating party* to the liaison (Myers, in *The Guardian*, 1 August 1989, my emphasis).

Feminists today continue to remain unclear about the kind of legal framework required. There are many dangers attendant on allying ourselves with the calls of the reactionary right for increased and tougher penalties. Revenge will not protect children. How can we best signal society's condemnation of abusers' actions, and minimize the risks of further abuse? Experience suggests that social workers should be very cautious about the possibility of effectively rehabilitating men who have perpetrated sexual offences against children (Dreiblatt 1982).

Victorian and early Edwardian perspectives on child sexual abuse may seem outdated, but at least they recognized its existence. How was it that child sexual abuse as a social issue disappeared for seventy years? The influence of Freud, whose personal volte-face on child sexual abuse has been widely analysed, is undoubtedly an important factor (Ward 1984; Miller 1985). Despite at first affirming the experiences of his middle-class female patients, Freud later asserted that they had 'fantasised' about the abuse by their fathers. A reassuring veil could thus be drawn across the possibility of 'ordinary' and 'respectable' fathers abusing their children.

The development of medical and pseudo-scientific models encouraged the notion that sexual offenders were 'mad' rather than 'bad' and hence absolved them of responsibility:

> Women's anger against men was deflated when responsibility was taken away from the male offender and attributed to his 'disease'. 'Sick' offenders could be seen as exceptions whose behaviour had little relevance to that of men in general (Jeffreys 1985: 85).

The portrayal of child sex abusers as victims of their own psychopathology ensured that ideals of the nuclear family would not be threatened. The advent of the era of so-called 'permissiveness' in the 1960s discouraged acknowledgement of the seamier sides of sexuality. The emergence of the paedophile movement in the 1970s further inhibited the recognition of child sexual abuse as a social problem and also strengthened the myth that homosexuals are paedophiles, and vice versa (McIntosh 1988). Heterosexual men whom, it has been estimated (Segal 1990), constitute the vast majority of abusers, were consequently shielded from public or professional attention.

By the late 1970s and early 1980s, however, women – via organizations such as Rape Crisis and Women's Aid – were developing a collective consciousness of the unrelenting dynamic of male violence in the family. Exposing the reality and extensiveness of child sexual abuse was an important part of this process. Feminists emphasized both the 'normalcy' of abuse, and the centrality of the dynamics of male power in the family in underpinning society's collusion with child sexual abuse.

Women experts in child sexual abuse have consistently been accused of attacking the basis of family life. There is more than a grain of truth in this accusation, as many feminists have cited the prevalence of child sexual abuse as a powerful argument in favour of their wider challenge to the conventional family. The feminist argument that child sexual abuse results from 'male supremacist attitudes and organisation, reinforced by the fundamental social structure of the family' (Ward 1984: 77) is rather disconcerting to supporters of traditional family values. Such criticisms of the family have been empirically substantiated by the thousands of women who have come forward in response to the publicity around child sexual abuse to disclose their own, long secret, experiences. Feminist perspectives had evidently struck a deep and profound chord with many women. The women's movement also raised questions about the values and methods of welfare professionals. However, the women's movement never anticipated how rapidly the issue of child sexual abuse would be taken over by a new welfare industry in which women's experiences and feminist perspectives would be marginalized.

The emergent child sexual abuse 'industry': are men in charge?

The concept of a child sexual abuse 'industry' might be regarded as diminishing the seriousness of sexual abuse. Yet a closer look at developments in late 1980s reveals that a whole new field of welfare has been established which appears to operate more in the interests of professionals than in the cause of survivors of child sexual abuse.

The recent expansion of child protection responsibilities has not been accompanied by an overall net expansion of welfare resources. 'New' resources for child sexual abuse have simply been transferred from other, less publicly visible, areas of welfare. Some additional funds for development, related to child sexual abuse have been made available by central government to local authorities, notably the Training Support Grants (Child Protection), sometimes known as 'post-Cleveland money'. But in few departments have there been any discernible increases in the numbers of front-line staff who are responsible for implementing child protection policies. Hence, while 'experts' (notably doctors and social work managers and academics) have been given the brief of producing 'solutions' to this new social problem, there has been no corresponding increase in the numbers of front-line staff who might implement any such 'solutions'. The MORI poll referred to earlier (Morris 1989) highlights the disjunction between the state's interest in being seen to be doing something about sexual abuse, and its preparedness to back this up with material resources for survivors.

One of the consequences of the displacement of feminism by welfare professionalism has been that the pivotal significance of gender politics and the patriarchal family in child sexual abuse has been undermined. The Cleveland inquiry report, for example, barely refers to the central relevance of gender and the maleness of most perpetrators. The denial of gender resulted from both the gradual ascendancy of a group of largely white middle-class male professional experts, and important shifts in the explanatory frameworks for child sexual abuse.

During the 1980s, white middle-class men, in their roles as gatekeepers of knowledge and as managers of welfare organizations, came to command the operations of this new 'industry' of child sexual abuse. This has encouraged white male ideas, rather than those of women or other disadvantaged groups, to prevail in professional and public discourses about child sexual abuse. Such developments have occurred despite the heavy reliance of welfare professionals on women's experiences and wisdom to lay bare the reality and meaning of such abuse. An example from television graphically illustrates the dominance of male voices in public discourses. In the *Testimony of a Child* debate on television, Esther Rantzen (TV presenter and co-founder of Childline) chaired a discussion about sexual abuse (BBC2 1989). Her panel comprised three male experts: David Mellor MP, David Tombs (Director of Social Services) and Dr Wyatt (one of the two paediatricians at the centre of the Cleveland crisis). Esther Rantzen apart, the only female voice was that of a adult survivor. It was clear that the woman survivor was there because of her experiences rather than because of any analysis she might offer. It was also significant that her husband was present at her side, implying that she could not be 'allowed' to speak autonomously.

Such images illustrate how women's voices have been deployed to make the issue visible, but also how they have been rapidly disempowered when it comes to analysing the problem and formulating and implementing policy. Kelly has commented:

> In the late 1980s it is the professionals and the state who are centre stage. We are on occasion credited with having raised the issues, but it is clearly now time for the 'real experts' to take over. This raises a series of contradictions for us, not to mention bitter ironies (Kelly 1989: 14).

Kelly points to the emergence of a male backlash against the feminist challenge over child sexual abuse. In the United States organizations have been formed with the primary purpose of defending men who are 'falsely accused' of child sexual abuse (Kelly 1989). There are, as yet, no British groups comparable to that of the American VOCAL (Victims of Child Abuse Laws) though Stuart Bell (Labour MP for Middlesbrough) took on this role in response to the Cleveland cases (Campbell 1988). Significant sectors of the press clearly share his approach. An article in the *Daily Mirror* the day after the publication of the report of the Cleveland inquiry detailed the 'bitterness' of parents whose 'lives were ruined in the Cleveland child-abuse scandal' (Crichmer, 7 July 1988). Such articles imply that it is the 'innocent' parents who were the true victims of the Cleveland crisis, rather than children who had been, or may have been, sexually abused. As Campbell has pointed out:

> The men's movement was classically populist – it articulated a revolt against professional power and yet it did so in the name not of the powerless – the children – but of the traditional authority of fathers within the family (Campbell 1988: 168).

By contrast, women 'experts' in child sexual abuse are presented as being either cold and calculating, or hysterical and emotional. This was all too apparent in the media's characterization of Dr Marietta Higgs (consultant paediatrician) and Sue Richardson (social worker) – the two central female professional figures in the Cleveland crisis. Both women became the targets of 'a massive and violent seizure of misogyny' (Nava 1988: 119); they were portrayed as insensitive figures whose feminist sympathies caused them to be over-zealous in removing children from their parents. Such media images diminish the seriousness and extensiveness of child sexual abuse.

In Britain it is noticeable that the 'big names' in child sexual abuse are predominantly male psychiatrists. Aarnon Bentovim, Tony Baker and Tilman Furniss are but three examples of men whose publications have had considerable influence on professional thinking. This is not to diminish the influence of a large number of female writers and researchers inside and outside social work. The writings of feminists such as Sarah Nelson (1987), Emily Driver (1989), and Beatrix Campbell (1988), for example, have been of great import in recasting ideas and practices. But, with the notable exception of Beatrix Campbell, such women are rarely afforded opportunities to appear in mainstream public and media debates. The fact that the men cited above hold prestigious posts in high-status academic or medical institutions is also important in conferring legitimacy on their opinions.

Although feminists have grown accustomed to hostile receptions to their ideas, the fury and distortion accompanying the backlash against feminist perspectives on child sexual abuse has been unprecedented. There have been overt condemnations and more subtle, but no less powerful, attempts to push feminists out of a central role in public debates. Women's incest survivors support groups have, for example, sometimes been at the receiving end of professional fears that such groups might indoctrinate the minds of survivors and thereby coerce them into being 'men haters' (Hudson 1985).

By the end of the 1980s, the idea that feminist perspectives might be 'extreme' and 'dangerous' had been semi-legitimated in professional social work literature. Kieran O'Hagan's work encapsulates this tendency in Britain. In the early pages of *Working with Child Sexual Abuse*, O'Hagan appears to acknowledge the importance of feminism in making the issue public. But later on, in a section entitled 'The extreme feminist view', he suggests there is a 'branch of feminism' that propagates:

> A view that *all* men are potential sexual abusers, *even of their own children*. Regrettably the hysteria and panic generated within social-services departments in recent years enabled this theory to become respectable and influential in social-work and feminist publications (O'Hagan 1989a: 98, his emphasis).

O'Hagan continues in this dismissive tone to argue that 'a pocketful of place-of-safety-orders' is all that is needed to put into practice such beliefs about child sexual abuse (O'Hagan 1989a: 98). Not only do such comments totally misrepresent feminist perspectives, they also imply that feminist social workers invoke their statutory powers without serious consideration of the implications for parental rights.

In the late 1980s, feminists challenged many of the premises of the family pathology approach to child sexual abuse. They confronted the idea that abuse was the consequence of distorted familial relationship patterns (see, for example, Porter 1984), because it diverted attention away from the overwhelming maleness of this form of abuse, and focused it instead on the culpability and collusiveness of mothers and daughters (Ward 1984; MacLeod and Saraga 1988a; Droisen and Driver 1989). Some feminist principles were taken on board by male experts and professionals; the importance of believing what children say and emphasizing that in no way is the abuse their fault or responsibility are obvious examples. Yet the acceptance of the relevance of issues of gender remained tokenistic, and was soon further undermined by the ascendancy of male experts and professional attitudes.

The prominence of the NSPCC as the national expert agency about sexual abuse is another indication of the power of male ideas and values. Some of its advertising messages, for example, suggest that men should have the monopoly where intervention with children who have been abused is concerned. In 1988 the NSPCC launched an appeal for funds for its £5 million Child Protection Training Centre in Leicester (opened in 1989). A press appeal showed a photograph of a young white female 'victim' in one corner of the advertisement. In another corner was a photograph of a slightly dishevelled looking white man, aged about thirty and wearing a jacket and tie with the top shirt button undone. Between the two photographs was the phrase 'She knows all about sexual abuse. Now we need to teach him' (*The Guardian* September 6, 1988). The message seemed clear enough: 'men know best' when it comes to supporting and protecting female 'victims'. What was somewhat perturbing and confusing, however, was that the image of the proposed male 'helper' was someone whose physical appearance looked stereotypically 'unsafe' and 'untrustworthy'.

The NSPCC has constantly needed to seek out new 'markets' in order to maintain its legitimacy and thereby to ensure its survival (Parton 1985). Its invitation to Mrs Thatcher to become vice-president in the late 1980s illustrates the Society's concern to maintain a high and politically acceptable public profile. The NSPCC has taken a lead role in promoting initiatives focused on child sexual abuse, many of which have made positive contributions to the development of practice wisdom. It has, for example, established specialist sexual abuse units, organized numerous conferences and training courses, and published an array of practice guidelines. Its high level of resources for staff training and for in-depth work with service users is often envied by those working in area social services teams. Yet a degree of caution is required in assessing the NSPCC contribution. First, despite the immediacy with which the NSPCC tends to be consulted in public debates about child abuse, it is local authorities who undertake the vast bulk of child abuse cases – approximately 95 per cent (Community Care 1989a). As such then, it is the latter who have the greatest body of first-hand experience of working with the complexities intrinsic to child sexual abuse work. Second, although the NSPCC possesses certain statutory child care powers, it only rarely works with a child throughout its career in the child care system. This may circumscribe its ability to comprehend the full implications of different methods of intervention.

At the heart of state-sponsored child protection work lies the issue of public intervention in the private arena of the family (Frost 1990). Unsurprisingly therefore, social work intervention involves almost irresolvable conflicts between protecting children and respecting the rights and civil liberties of parents. Dingwall *et al.* (1983) have argued that there can be no technical solution to the complex moral and political issues raised by child protection work. Society ultimately has to calculate 'How much freedom is a child's life worth?' (Dingwall *et al.* 1983: 244). The Cleveland crisis confirmed that the state regards it as more important that the authority of fathers is upheld than children protected from sexual abuse. The media's blanket of silence on questions of familial power and gender politics reinforced this approach (Nava 1988).

By contrast, inquiries into the deaths of Jasmine Beckford and Kimberley Carlile (London Borough of Brent 1985; London Borough of Greenwich 1987) drew attention to the failure of social workers and allied professionals to enforce statutory powers. As Franklin has pointed out, press coverage of these cases 'lampooned social workers as indecisive wimps'; yet only a few months later, when events in Cleveland came to dominate the press, 'the target remained the same but the imagery was reversed and the social worker emerged as the authoritarian bully' (Franklin 1989: 5). It can surely be no coincidence that the social worker appears as a 'wimp' in instances involving physical abuse, while being depicted as a 'bully' attacking family life in situations involving sexual abuse.

Reclaiming feminist principles in social work practice

Feminist social work is always fraught with challenges and contradictions, but nowhere is this more apparent than in the field of sexual abuse. How do we attain the best possible balance between parental liberties and child protection? Is the removal of a child from his or her family always the most appropriate response to the disclosure of sexual abuse? There are no simple answers to these questions, yet they daily confront practitioners and their managers. This section explores some of the practice implications of the male-centred perspectives that have come to dominate child sexual abuse work in Britain, and considers how we might begin to reclaim feminist principles in practice.

The Cleveland inquiry report focused more on the recognition and investigation of child sexual abuse than on practical methods of tackling the problem. The report recommended close inter-agency cooperation, warned against the 'danger of false identification' and called for more staff training. The inquiry's almost obsessive focus on the diagnosis of abuse diverted attention away from what should be done after a positive disclosure has been made. But apart from considering changes in the legal framework and emphasizing the importance of parents being able to participate in decision-making processes, it had little to say about the constituents of 'good practice' after a disclosure had been made.

Though the state insists on the importance of child protection, it refuses to place a priority on providing resources and services for children who are at risk. Though Mrs Thatcher reassured children 'don't hesitate to phone' the Childline service, she did not provide more funds for agencies who follow up appeals for help (*P.M.* BBC Radio Four, 31 May 1990).

The central, rather limited, goal of local-authority based child protection work is often to ensure that a child is not subject to abuse or neglect. In this respect the modern social worker operates like a Victorian social purity campaigner engaged in 'saving' children from a life of vice. Once a child has been admitted to care following disclosures of sexual abuse, social workers feel that they can breathe a sigh of relief, since the child can be deemed to be 'safe'. Many children and young people are then effectively neglected through professional inaction and lack of resources. The emphasis on diagnosis and investigation has rendered post-validation work with children and young people, and their non-abusing parents as something of an extra to be served out only in meagre portions. This policy is tantamount to the secondary abuse of children who have already been abused.

The Cleveland report emphasized the need for agencies to build up professional expertise, and to ensure that they established 'structured arrangements for their professional supervision and personal support' (HMSO 1988: 247). But supervisory practices in most social work agencies remain unsatisfactory, and many managers still lack the requisite skills and knowledge. The post-Cleveland child protection training grants have opened up training opportunities for practitioners and their managers. But the small amounts of money involved, together with the large numbers of staff who require such training, have greatly circumscribed the impact of these initiatives.

It is well known that institutions often organize structured defence systems to cope with the anxiety implicit in a particular role or task (Menzies 1970). The near obsession with procedures in dealing with child sexual abuse in many statutory agencies suggests that these are a form of defence against the full recognition of the emotional and political meaning of sexual abuse. As Sue Richardson has pointed out, child sexual abuse is not 'necessarily amenable to straightforward problem-solving' (Richardson 1989: 121). 'Checklists' of 'risk factors' which are supposed to predict which children might be at risk of abuse may allow social workers and allied professionals to feel more comfortable, but they do not necessarily accurately 'predict' which children will be abused. The assumption that procedures or checklists in themselves will protect children is obviously illusory.

Given the mystification of child sexual abuse by many professional experts in the 'industry', it is important to insist that the basic principles and skills involved are fairly straightforward, and in fact are already well understood by many social workers. The idea that 'only experts should do this work' has often undermined the confidence and competence of 'ordinary' front-line practitioners, most of whom are women. Those who are already experienced in other forms of child care work, such as working with children in care and undertaking preventive work with children and families, will often have the skills of sensitive communication with children and young people, of assessment, and of planning and structuring their work.

The work of Rape Crisis centres, Women's Aid and incest survivors' groups have all revealed the power of collective sharing of women's experience of male violence (MacLeod and Saraga 1988b). The idea that (predominantly female) front-line social workers need to receive lengthy training at the feet of 'real' experts before they can undertake work with survivors of sexual abuse denies the validity of women's experiences, and undervalues the major contribution the women's movement has made to the whole field of child sexual abuse. Driver has pointed out that women have the potential for skills that male experts may never learn:

> Our forgotten ability to empathise with the child, to study the options that children have and to try to learn from the ways in which they themselves deploy those options. In taking the child's eye view on sexual abuse, we have to unlearn many of our adult assumptions about the phenomenon (Driver 1989: 173).

The concern of many white feminists to ensure that issues of child sexual abuse are placed at the heart of the social work agenda has eclipsed the equally important imperative of linking issues about the power of gender in families with those relating to race, class and sexual identity. Social work has a long way to go before its child protection duties are executed in a socially equitable way. It is significant that the Cleveland inquiry report made no specific mention of the needs of different racial groups among social services consumers. Few articles and books about sexual abuse have addressed the impact of race, racism and culture. Similarly, social services departments have been inconsistent in implementing anti-discrimination policies relating to child sexual abuse. Islington social services department is one of the relatively few agencies which has made explicit the importance of social workers' taking account of the impact of racism and of cultural factors in assessment and intervention in child sexual abuse work (Boulshel and Noakes 1988).

Black children who are being sexually abused are subject to racialized images of sexual abuse that may make the process of disclosure even more difficult. Contemporary stereotypes present conflicting images of black children and child sexual abuse. On the one hand such abuse is presented as 'white problems' (Bogle 1988: 134), because of the consistent omission of black children from discussion. On the other hand, however, sexual abuse is also frequently portrayed as normative in black people's cultures. This is illustrated in the following quote from a social worker (taken from my research about young women in trouble):

> '[He is] half Jamaican, half Chinese . . . he was brought up by his grandmother and he hated his mother. I think . . . that may well lead to the *very different view of sexual norms*' (a social worker talking about the father of a young woman in care who had recently disclosed sexual abuse by the former; my emphasis).

Such views reflect the racist idea that child sexual abuse is an accepted component of 'ethnic minority' cultures (Ahmad 1989: 34). They further perpetuate pathological stereotypes of black families and they carry the danger that black children who are being abused will remain vulnerable as a result of professional inaction. Social workers' fear of being perceived as racist may mean that many white professionals 'shy away from their duties of protecting the black child from abuse' (Ahmad 1989). The hesitation to intervene may put some children from black families at considerable risk (Channer and Parton 1990) and imply that black children have fewer rights than their white counterparts.

A number of issues must be kept at the forefront when working with black children and their families. First, black children may find it particularly difficult to speak of their experiences of sexual abuse to the white employees of social services departments. As with other forms of domestic violence, fear of the police and state intervention makes black women reluctant to seek either police or social work help (MacLeod and Saraga 1988a; Mama 1990). The older the child, the greater the likelihood that they will be aware of the potential repercussions of police involvement and the greater the reluctance to disclose abuse. Joan Riley's novel *The Unbelonging* offers a powerful and poignant account of the dilemmas faced by a young black 11-year-old who wants to escape the abuse and violence of her father, but who also greatly fears the intervention of white law and order:

> She knew that she did not need money to phone the police, just had to dial 999; but the thought of doing that frightened her almost as much as going back. 'They don't like neaga here'. The words came back to her, echoing in her head every time she tried to build up the courage to make the call (Riley 1985: 63–4).

In most areas of the country it is now policy for the police and social services staff to undertake joint investigations. This has undoubtedly had many positive benefits, but it may also exacerbate the stress of disclosure for black children. Most children who have been sexually abused feel a deep sense of guilt, and they often retain a strong loyalty to the perpetrators of the abuse. Black children's sense of 'betrayal' may be particularly strong given the repressive consequences of disclosure. The situation is also particularly difficult for black mothers. As Bogle has pointed out:

> Black women, in trying to protect their own children, face racism from the police which can compound the abuse already suffered by the children (Bogle 1988: 134).

The disclosure of sexual abuse may lead to the dissolution of both black and white family networks. But the loss of familial support may be particularly distressing and damaging to a black child, when the alternatives provided are white dominated. As Droisen has pointed out, 'Children protect their communities. They don't want to add fuel to the fire of prejudice' (Droisen 1989: 163). In Asian communities the stigma of a 'violated female' child within the family may mean that the children are considered 'no longer marriageable' (Mtezuka 1989–90).

The disadvantages incurred by black children are further compounded if they are admitted to local authority care. Black children, for example, seem more likely to spend longer periods of time in care (Channer and Parton 1990). A Commission for Racial Equality survey in 1988 found that only a few social services departments have race equality policies which take explicit account of the needs of black and ethnic minority children in care (Commission for Racial Equality 1990). The Children Act 1989 is the first piece of child care legislation to make explicit reference to the duty of local authorities to take account of a child's cultural, religious, racial and linguistic background in its decision making processes (see Langan in this volume). We have yet to see what kind of impact the Act will have on the shape and quality of child care services to black and ethnic minority children.

Though it has long been recognized that child sexual abuse occurs in all social classes, working-class families are much more likely to become the target of official intervention. This is because they are subject to more intensive social policing, through the intervention of social workers, health visitors and teachers. Prejudiced assumptions that child sexual abuse is common in working-class communities are thereby perpetuated and fuelled. O'Hagan's writing provides evidence of such beliefs:

> Most social workers are daily immersed in the dilapidated sprawling council estates and disintegrating communities of

> fragmented families, the offices in which they work are inundated with child sexual abuse referrals from such localities (O'Hagan 1989b: 13).

There is also a well-established prejudice that children are more at risk from gay men than from heterosexual men. The 'public terror' about homosexual men corrupting minors stands in significant contrast to the near total lack of outrage about the sexually abusive acts of heterosexual men (Segal 1990: 159). So, although society is now having to face the fact that heterosexual men abuse girls and young women, gay men and lesbians continue to be vulnerable to assumptions that they are potentially 'dangerous' where work with children and young people is concerned (see Brown in this volume).

The sexual abuse of boys and young men presents some complex practice dilemmas. The law defines sexual contact between a 21-year-old man and a 16-year-old man as abusive. In some situations this may be an appropriate definition, for example where financial and other forms of exploitation are concerned. In others, however, the instigation of a child sexual abuse investigation will convey negative messages about homosexuality to the young person involved.

All of those working with survivors of child sexual abuse must remain open to the need to revise and shift our understandings and practice. An obvious illustration of this relates to the possibility of women sexually abusing children. We cannot afford to presume that this is an impossibility. When children have disclosed sexual abuse by female adults we must take care neither to excuse nor rationalize such abuse. Nor should we resort to pathological explanations, since this would be to replicate the criticisms made by feminists of traditional male perspectives on sexual abuse.

Some commentators have seized on the undeniable reality that there are some female perpetrators of child sexual abuse to refute the centrality of gender. Erin Pizzey, whose perspectives on domestic violence have often been the focus of feminist criticism, has commented:

> I believe that the time has come for us to put aside the assumption that all issues of abuse are issues of gender (Pizzey 1990).

The socially constructed dynamics of gender lie at the heart of our sexual practice. Women, no less than men, are subject to absorbing particular meanings about sexuality. Although women are less likely to associate sexuality with violence, for some women the link between domination, power and sexuality may result in the sexual abuse of children. Though we are still at an early stage in understanding why some women sexually abuse children, we cannot afford to evade the issue. To do so will not only play into the hands of those who want to discredit feminist perspectives, more importantly, it will harm those children who have been abused by women.

Child sexual abuse brings into relief the sometimes conflicting objectives of protecting women and children from male familial power, while seeking to minimize the state's potential to erode further the rights and liberties of disadvantaged groups and communities. For example, should the police share information about unsuccessful convictions of an adult for sexual assault on children? Some might argue that the disclosure of such information is inequitable, given that there has been a finding of not guilty, and would result in unjust and unaccountable social work decision-making. Others, however, would argue that the very considerable difficulties in obtaining 'satisfactory' evidence means that only a minority of such offenders are ever found guilty. The interests of protecting children are regarded as overriding the need to defend adults' civil liberties.

The Cleveland inquiry highlighted the fact that the removal of children to the presumed safety of local authority care does not guarantee children the support to which they should have a right. But where the inquiry made a fundamental error was in subsuming parents in one catch-all category; both the inquiry and much press coverage of child sexual issues has failed to differentiate between mothers and fathers. The rights and needs of abusing parents are surely very different from those of non-abusing parents. It is significant that Sue Richardson's one source of regret about the Cleveland crisis was that no one empowered mothers (Campbell 1988: 165).

In many respects, the recognition of the extensiveness of child sexual abuse as a feature of the lives of many social services users and providers has created the opportunity for the development of more sensitive responses to social work consumers. Our comprehension of some of the issues facing, for example, 'runaway' young women and adult women who constantly feel depressed has been greatly enhanced by knowledge and understanding about child sexual abuse. After a rather halting start, social workers have begun to attempt to define 'good practice' (see, for example, Glaser and Frosh 1988; MacLeod and Saraga 1988b). But definitions of 'good practice' do not evolve in a vacuum; they are shaped and moulded by complex, and often opposing, political and professional interests. This chapter has sought to show that it is imperative that some brakes are put on the move towards the creation of a welfare industry which seeks to advance professional interests rather than those of child and adult survivors of sexual abuse.

References

Ahmad, B. (1989), 'Protecting black children from abuse', *Social Work Today* 8 June, p. 24.

Bailey, S. and Blackburn, N. (1979), 'The Punishment of Incest Act 1908: A case study of law creation', *Criminal Law Review* pp. 702–12.

Bogle, M. T. (1988), 'Brixton black women's centre: organizing on child sexual abuse', *Feminist Review* 28, pp. 132–5.

Boulshel, M. and Noakes, S. (1988), 'Islington social services: developing a policy on child sexual abuse', *Feminist Review* 28, pp. 150–7.

Campbell, B. (1988), *Unofficial Secrets* (London: Virago).

Channer, Y. and Parton, N. (1990), 'Racism, cultural relativism and child protection', in The Violence Against Children Study Group, *Taking Child Abuse Seriously* (London: Unwin Hyman) pp. 105–20.

Commission for Racial Equality (1990), *Adopting a Better Policy: Adoption and Fostering of Ethnic Minority Children* (London: Commission for Racial Equality).

Community Care (1989a), 'News', *Community Care* 20 April.

Community Care (1989b), 'Survey to show growth in child abuse cases', *Community Care* 3 August.

Crichmer, C. (1988), 'So what happens to us now?' *Daily Mirror* 7 July.

Dingwall, R., Eekelaar, J. and Murray, T. (1983), *The Protection of Children: State Intervention and Family Life* (Oxford: Basil Blackwell).

Donzelot, J. (1980), *The Policing of Families* (London: Hutchinson).

Dreiblatt, I. (1982), *Issues in the Evaluation of the Sex Offender* Washington State Psychological Association Meeting, May.

Driver, E. (1989), 'Introduction', in E. Driver and A. Droisen (eds), 1989.

Driver, E. and Droisen, A. (eds) (1989), *Child Sexual Abuse: Feminist Perspectives* (Basingstoke: Macmillan).

Droisen, A. (1989), 'Racism and anti-racism' in E. Driver and A. Droisen, 1989, pp. 158–69.

Franklin, B. (1989), 'Wimps and bullies: press reporting of child abuse', in B. Carter, T. Jeffs and M. Smith (eds), *Social Work and Social Policy Yearbook 1* (Milton Keynes: Open University Press) pp. 1–14.

Frost, N. (1990), 'Official intervention and child protection: the relationship between state and family in contemporary Britain', in The Violence Against Children Study Group, *Taking Child Abuse Seriously* (London: Unwin Hyman) pp. 25–40.

Glaser, D. and Frosh, S. (1988), *Child Sexual Abuse* (Basingstoke: Macmillan).

Gordon, L. (1989), *Heroes of Their Own Lives* (London: Virago).

HMSO (1988), *Report of the Inquiry into Child Abuse in Cleveland* (London: HMSO).

Hudson, A. (1985), 'Feminism and social work: resistance or dialogue?', *British Journal of Social Work* 15, pp. 635–55.

Jeffreys, S. (1985), *The Spinster and Her Enemies* (London: Pandora).

Jones, C. (1983), *State Social Work and the Working Class* (Basingstoke: Macmillan).

Kelly, L. (1989), 'Bitter ironies; the professionalisation of child abuse', *Trouble and Strife* 16, pp. 14–21.

London Borough of Brent (1985), *A Child in Trust: Report of the Panel of Inquiry Investigating the Circumstances Surrounding the Death of Jasmine Beckford* (London Borough of Brent).

London Borough of Greenwich (1987), *A Child in Mind: Protection of Children in a Responsible Society: Report of the Commission of Inquiry surrounding the death of Kimberley Carlile* (London Borough of Greenwich).

MacLeod, M. and Saraga, E. (1988a), 'Challenging the orthodoxy: towards a feminist theory and practice', *Feminist Review* 28, pp. 16–55.

MacLeod, M. and Saraga, E. (eds) (1988b), *Child Sexual Abuse: Towards a Feminist Professional Practice*, Report of a conference held at the Polytechnic of North London (London: Polytechnic of North London).

McIntosh, M. (1988), 'Introduction to an issue: family secrets as public drama', *Feminist Review* 28, pp. 6–15.

Mama, A. (1990), *The Hidden Struggle* (London: London Race and Housing Research Unit and the Runnymede Trust).

Menzies, I. (1970), *The Functioning of Social Systems as a Defence against Anxiety* (London: The Tavistock Institute for Human Relations).

Miller, A. (1985), *Thou Shalt Not be Aware* (London: Pluto).

Morris, P. (1989), 'No let up after Cleveland', *Community Care*, 1 June, p. 7.

Mtezuka, M. (1989–90), 'Towards a better understanding of child sexual abuse among Asian communities' (Manchester: in *Practice*, nos 3–4. School of Social Work, University of Manchester).

Myers, P. (1989), 'Appeal carer doubles incest case sentence', *The Guardian*, 1 August.

Nava, M. (1988), 'Cleveland and the press: outrage and anxiety in the reporting of child sexual abuse' *Feminist Review* 28, pp. 103–21.

Nelson, S. (1987), *Incest: Fact and Myth* (Edinburgh: Stramullion).

O'Hagan, K. (1989a), *Working with Child Sexual Abuse* (Milton Keynes: Open University Press).

O'Hagan, K. (1989b), 'Split decisions prevent progress', *Community Care* 9 March, p. 13.

Parton, N. (1985), *The Politics of Child Abuse* (Basingstoke: Macmillan).
Pizzey, E. (1990), 'Child abuse by both sexes', letter in *The Independent*, June 7.
Porter, R. (ed.) (1984), *Child Sexual Abuse Within the Family* (London: Tavistock/CIBA Foundation).

Richardson, S. (1989), 'Child sexual abuse: the challenge for the organization', in P. Carter, T. Jeffs and M. Smith (eds), *Social Work and Social Welfare* (Milton Keynes: Open University Press) pp. 118–28.
Riches, V. (1990), 'Break-up of family unit puts children in danger', *The Independent*, 28 April.
Riley, J. (1985), *The Unbelonging* (London: The Women's Press).

Satyamurti, C. (1979), 'Care and control in local authority social work', in N. Parry, M. Rustin and C. Satyamurti, *Social Work, Welfare and the State* (London: Edward Arnold).
Segal, L. (1990), *Slow Motion: Changing Masculinities, Changing Men* (London: Virago).

Viinikka, S. (1989), 'Child sexual abuse and the law', in E. Driver and A. Droisen (eds), *Child Sexual Abuse* (Basingstoke: Macmillan).

Ward, E. (1984), *Father Daughter Rape* (London: The Women's Press).
Weeks, J. (1981), *Sex, Politics and Society* (London: Hutchinson).
Wohl, A. S. (1970), 'Introduction', in A. S. Wohl (ed.), *Bitter Cry of Outcast London* (Leicester: Leicester University Press).
Wohl, A. S. (1978), 'Sex and the single room: incest among the Victorian working classes', in A. S. Wohl (ed.), *The Victorian Family* (London: Croom Helm).
Woodcraft (1988), 'Child sexual abuse and the law', *Feminist Review* 28, pp. 122–30.

8 *Women with learning difficulties are women too*

Fiona Williams

Introduction

Over the last decade or so, there has been increasing acknowledgement of the fact that people with learning difficulties constitute one of the most marginalized and oppressed groups in society. People labelled as 'mentally handicapped' have often been denied the right to integrate with others, the right to marry, the right to parenthood, the right to vote, the right to freedom from harassment, violence and abuse (Ryan and Thomas 1987). Many people with learning difficulties are denied paid work, or else are highly exploited in the paid work they do (Wertheimer 1981), and they often experience substantial poverty (Sumpton 1988; Flynn 1989). Their behaviour is often stereotyped in devaluing, negative and often contradictory ways – as child-like, dangerous, promiscuous, volatile or insensible (Wolfensberger 1975). Furthermore, many state policies and institutional practices continue to intensify some of these aspects of oppression (Tyne 1982).

At the same time, however, significant challenges to these processes of marginalization and oppression have emerged. Policies of de-institutionalization and community care have long received official support, though the resources to ensure the success of these policies have been less forthcoming (Walker 1982). More significant are the challenges that have come from local initiatives (Shearer 1986), from pressure groups (such as CMH – Campaign for Valued Futures with People who have Learning Difficulties), from researchers (Towell 1988) and not least from people with learning difficulties themselves. The strategy of 'normalization', endorsed by many campaigners, has sought to provide ways for people with learning difficulties to integrate into the mainstream of society, to participate and be valued members of society and enjoy the same rights, opportunities and patterns of living as others in society (Nirje 1970; O'Brien and Tyne 1981; Wolfensberger 1972; 1983).

In addition, the development of advocacy and self-advocacy groups has been important in providing ways of empowering people with learning difficulties (for example, the People First movement; see Williams and Schoultz 1982; Crawley 1988). There have also been initiatives in non-institutional forms of community living in which people with learning difficulties have some control over how they want to live their lives (Shearer 1986; Ward 1988; Towell 1988). Strategies such as 'individual programme planning' and 'shared action planning' have attempted to acknowledge the diversity of individual needs and create ways in which these can be expressed, for example, by encouraging more equal and cooperative relationships between service users and providers (Blunden 1980; Open University 1986; 1990; Brechin and Swain 1987).

A new set of concerns has emerged from these developments. Workers and researchers in this field have come to recognize that while people with learning difficulties are oppressed, they are not necessarily a homogeneous group. Their interests and needs are different, not just because they have different degrees of disability, but because they are divided in terms of class, race, gender and age.[1] How significant are these divisions among people with learning difficulties? What effects do they have on the provision of services? Do they generate compounded inequalities? Are experiences of oppression doubled or even tripled? What strategies exist for practitioners and for people with learning difficulties themselves to overcome these inequalities? How do these issues affect strategies such as 'normalization'?

This chapter will explore these issues in relation to women with learning difficulties, taking into account the fact that the experiences and life chances of women are themselves differentiated by race and class divisions. These are relatively under-researched areas, and the following discussion is a tentative exploration of some of the complex issues affecting people with learning difficulties.

Converging stereotypes

Negative stereotyping is a common element in the process of marginalization and subordination suffered by oppressed groups – women, black people, the poor, disabled people. However, what is particularly significant for women who have learning difficulties is that many of the stereotypes about people with learning difficulties *converge with* sexist and racist stereotyping. So, for example, both women and people with learning difficulties are widely considered to be irrational, submissive, volatile, passive, manipulative, unable to make their own choices or decisions, excitable and possessed of a hidden but dangerous sexuality. Like most stereotypes, these include contradictory elements: women and people with learning difficulties are characterized as *both* submissive and dangerous, *both* irrational and cunning, *both* innocent and tainted. Both virgin and whore; both holy innocent and social menace. Helen Smith and Hilary Brown suggest that the parallels between the experiences of women and people with mental disabilities (both mental illness and mental handicap), give rise to a common sense of powerlessness, dependence and 'otherness' (Smith and Brown 1989).

Carole Baxter has pointed to the similarities between the stereotyping of people with learning difficulties and of black and minority ethnic groups (Baxter 1989). She draws on seminal work by Wolf Wolfensberger (1975) in which he identifies eight 'negative social roles' which have been attributed to people with learning difficulties: subhuman; sick; holy innocent; eternal child; object of pity and burden of charity; object of ridicule; menace; and object of dread. Baxter argues that these are the ways in which black people have traditionally been stereotyped, and they have provided the justifications for their continued oppression. Thus for example, the stereotyping of people with learning difficulties as a menace has led in the past to their being institutionalized and sexually segregated to prevent them from having children and contaminating the 'national stock'. Local communities still object to residential services for people with learning difficulties being sited in their neighbourhoods on the spurious grounds of the potential danger they represent. Baxter compares this with the ways in which black communities in Britain have been subjected to more repressive policing, and their over-representation in prisons and in mental hospitals. Black cultures too are often represented as a threat to 'traditional British values' (Hall *et al.* 1978). Such stereotyping leads both black people and people with learning difficulties to become the victims of physical harassment, abuse and ridicule.

A further example is the portrayal of black people as 'eternal children' requiring control, management and spiritual guidance from their white 'superiors', a notion which became one of the justifications for colonialism and imperialism. Similarly adult people with learning difficulties are often treated as perpetual children. They are referred to as having a 'mental age' of six or seven, without any acknowledgement of their emotional maturity; they are given pocket money rather than wages; they are dressed in short white socks and sandals.

Following Baxter's observation that racist images can acquire an additional intensity when attributed to black people with learning difficulties, we can suggest that the convergence of sexist and racist stereotypes with stereotypes of people with learning difficulties becomes particularly poignant for women with learning difficulties, and even more so for black women with learning difficulties.

However, it would be a mistake to push the comparisons between different forms of oppression too far. The oppressions of sex, race and mental handicap have different histories, different roots and different paths. This is so even though the processes which render white or black women or women with learning difficulties subordinate may appear similar, and may give rise to the possibility of a shared understanding between these groups. What is significant is that the lives of women with learning difficulties are structured through mental (and sometimes physical) disability, as well as through gender and class, and, for black women with learning difficulties, additionally through race. These simultaneous experiences do not just operate in parallel forms, but they compound and reconstitute the experience of oppression for women with learning difficulties in very specific ways. This is particularly the case when the stereotypes converge around specific themes like dependence or sexuality. For example, rights to motherhood are granted to some women (able-bodied, respectable white women) but not fully to others (black women, poor women, Third World women) and hardly at all to others (women with learning difficulties, black or white).

A second point arises from these observations about converging stereotypes. The overlap of stereotypes between people with learning difficulties, women and black people has led at times to the over-representation of these groups among those defined as 'mentally handicapped'. Indeed, this overlapping of stereotypes demonstrates the extent to which definitions of mental handicap are as much social constructions based upon existing social divisions as they are definitions of perceptible intellectual impairments. Take, for example, the construction of 'mental deficiency' in Britain in the early part of this century.

The 1913 Mental Deficiency Act, one of the first major pieces of state intervention for people with learning difficulties, graded them as 'mentally deficient', 'idiots', 'imbeciles' or 'feeble-minded', and approved the detention of many of those so-labelled in institutions. Here they were separated from their families and from society, and, more importantly in terms of the aims of the act, separated from the opposite sex. These aims reflected a concern to protect people with learning difficulties from exploitation, neglect and ill-treatment in the outside world. But they also reflected a concern to protect the outside world from the social, moral and 'racial' threat which people with learning difficulties were seen to represent.

The issue of mental deficiency generated a moral panic, centring upon feeble-minded women. Writing in 1912, W. E. Fernald, superintendent of the Massachusetts School for the Feeble-minded from 1887 to 1924, revealed the prevailing prejudices:

> Feeble-minded women are almost invariably immoral and if at large usually become carriers of disease or give birth to children who are as defective as themselves. The feeble-minded woman who marries is twice as prolific as the normal woman (quoted in Abbott and Sapsford 1987: 25).

The stereotypes of feeble-minded women as immoral, carriers of venereal disease, bearers of defective children, promiscuous, over-fertile and a cause of potential social, economic and moral decline dominated official policy. Such ideas were sustained by the specious scientific arguments of the eugenics movement, which emphasized the importance of heredity in reproducing mental deficiency. Authorities firmly believed that the incidence of mental deficiency was much greater in certain social groups – among the poor and unskilled working-class, and immigrant groups. These beliefs were reinforced by influential theories about a supposed hierarchy of races, with the white races at the top and the black races at the bottom. Such ideas were also reflected in medical views about women. The study by Ehrenreich and English of medical practice in the early-twentieth century shows how doctors stereotyped upper-class and working-class women in different ways. Upper-class women were seen as weak, inherently sick, given to hysteria and capable of only leisurely pastimes. By contrast, poor working-class, black and immigrant women were seen, on the one hand as strong and robust, and on the other as a threat to the race, overbreeding and harbouring disease (Ehrenreich and English 1976). Since the stereotypes about feeble-mindedness overlapped so much with views of poor working-class women, it is not surprising to find that many more women than men were detained in institutions. For example, in 1932 in the Meanwood Park Colony in Leeds more than 60 per cent of the residents were women – 263 women and 160 men (City of Leeds 1932). Although sex differences in intellectual impairments is a little researched area, contemporary figures for the United States show that they are more prevalent amongst men than amongst women (Alexander *et al.* 1985).

While it would be wrong to suggest that negative stereotypes were carried wholesale into policy, nevertheless, a second example from post-war Britain illustrates the way in which racist stereotyping converged with definitions about subnormality. In the 1960s, a disproportionate number of Afro-Caribbean school-children were labelled as 'Educationally Sub-Normal' (ESN). Afro-Caribbean mothers have given their account of this practice in *Heart of the Race*:

> It was the attitude of the teachers that did the most lasting damage. They were to interpret Black children's disorientation and

> bewilderment as a sign of stupidity. Their concepts of us as simple-minded, happy folk, lacking in sophistication or sensitivity, became readily accepted definitions. Theories about us, put forward by Jenson in America and endorsed by Eysenck here in the late sixties gave such views a spurious credibility by popularising the idea that race and intelligence are linked in some inherent way . . . Because of such reactions, we came to be labelled as 'dull' and 'disruptive' (Bryan, Dadzie and Scafe 1985: 64–5).

This inappropriate labelling of Afro-Caribbean children as ESN reveals how the historical legacy of a 'hierarchy of races' reappeared in more refined theoretical reformulations about race and intelligence. It also shows the ways in which racist stereotypes about black children, black families and black cultures overlapped with prevalent definitions of subnormality.

The areas of sexuality and reproduction show the impact of converging stereotypes upon the lives and experiences of women with learning difficulties.

Reproductive rights and sexuality

> People like us don't have babies. No one in the centre does apart from the staff. Some people have their stomachs taken out (woman with learning difficulties quoted in Atkinson and Williams 1990: 175).

Many, if not most, women with learning difficulties do not have children. In the case of many severely handicapped women, especially in institutions, opportunities to develop sexual relationships are restricted. Some women with specific types of impairment may have reduced fertility (National Institute on Mental Retardation (NIMR) 1980); some women may choose not to have children, others may have this choice made for them. In particular, carers or local authorities may decide on behalf of a woman with learning difficulties that she should be sterilized.

In the past, the 'problem' of the sexuality of women with learning difficulties was resolved by institutionalization and segregation. However, with the move towards community care, more local authorities and parents have been requesting, through the courts, for the right to decide upon sterilization on behalf of their client or daughter. Those who defend the decision to sterilize in these circumstances generally do so on the grounds that it offers protection to the woman from the traumas of pregnancy and childbirth and from the responsibilities of child-rearing. Sterilization is also justified as an effective form of contraception; more radical surgery also eliminates the need for menstrual care.

The sterilization of women without their direct consent raises important questions about the terms upon which society will admit people with learning difficulties into the mainstream. Does it mean that the granting of rights in one area – the right to live in the community and develop relationships – carries with it the denial of rights in another area – the rights to reproduction and motherhood? Sterilization also raises questions about the assumptions upon which decisions are taken – assumptions about the sexuality of women with learning difficulties, about who are and who are not 'unfit mothers', indeed what constitutes an 'unfit baby'. These are not just 'mental handicap' issues, they also raise gender, race and class questions. In addition, sterilization raises questions about who makes the decision, and whether less invasive strategies are available.

Assessments about women's capacity to understand their sexuality and the possibilities of conception are often based on the woman's 'mental age'. One widely publicized case was that of 'Jeanette' a 17-year-old girl with Down's Syndrome who was sterilized without her own consent following hearings in the Appeal Court and the House of Lords in 1987, in response to requests from the local authority and her mother. Jeanette was said to have a 'mental age' of five or six. However, such 'mental ages' are often based on cognitive skills rather than emotional capacities, or even emotional potential. It is significant that in Jeanette's case what had precipitated the action by her mother and the local authority was the fact that Jeanette was showing signs of sexual awareness and sexual drive 'with a risk of pregnancy' (Cawson 1987), revealing, perhaps, emotional maturity far beyond that of a 6-year-old.

Such concern that a woman's growing sexual awareness might lead to pregnancy may be based on hidden assumptions about either potential promiscuity, or extreme passive vulnerability. In fact, Jeanette spent her weekdays in local authority care and her weekends at home; she did not use public transport, nor had she money of her own to spend. She had, in fact, little opportunity to 'risk' pregnancy. This is not to underestimate the vulnerability of women like Jeanette to sexual abuse, nor to underestimate their carers' anxiety about this (Brown and Craft 1989). However, sterilization does not itself solve the problem of sexual vulnerability even though it removes the associated risk of pregnancy. One problem, therefore, with granting the right to sterilize without direct consent is that such action may reinforce old stereotypes about the fertility and sexual proclivities of women with learning difficulties.

Another question raised by the issue of sterilization is the capacity of women with learning difficulties for motherhood. It is often assumed that a woman's right to conceive is sacrosanct, but in fact policies and practices in relation to contraception, abortion and in vitro fertilization (IVF) reveal that women with learning difficulties are not the only group often considered to be 'unfit' to bear children. The imposition of contraception, like the long-lasting drug Depo-Provera, or even enforced sterilization and abortion upon black and poor white women in both the Third World and the West, reveals pressures to discourage the fertility of certain groups of women. The guidelines proposed in the 1985 Warnock Report on the use of infertility treatments such as IVF, egg and embryo donation and artificial insemination, suggested that these should be restricted to women living in stable heterosexual relationships (Stanworth 1987). All this suggests that there is a hierarchy of eligibility for motherhood in which women with learning difficulties are at the bottom and white respectable able-bodied women at the top. Given the intermediate position of black women then it could be assumed that this position would be compounded for black women with learning difficulties.

There has been little research into the fact that few women with learning difficulties have or care for children. To what extent do these women decide for themselves not to have children, or respond to negative evaluations of their capacity for motherhood? How far, given support and development of skills, could women with learning difficulties achieve their aspirations? How far does the low socio-economic position of women with learning difficulties reinforce the concept of them as 'unfit mothers'? It is important to disentangle the general social and economic situation of women with learning difficulties from their capacity to mother. Many people with learning difficulties who live independently also live in poverty (Flynn 1989). Indeed, it is an irony that people whose capacities for normal living are considered to be limited are put to the exacting test of surviving on minimal state benefits, a task requiring great skills in budgeting, thrift and the exercise of welfare rights. They often have little social support and suffer harassment from neighbours (Flynn 1989). Parenthood in these conditions would prove taxing even for somebody without learning difficulties.

A further issue which follows on from the discussion of 'unfit mothers' is that of the 'unfit baby'. How far does the screening of pregnant women for foetal abnormalities reinforce the devaluation of people with learning difficulties and disabled people?

Genetic screening gives mothers, or parents, an opportunity to decide whether they feel able to care for a child with disabilities, and if they do, to prepare for that. Some disabled women have, however, argued that one of the assumptions underlying such testing is that mothers want only 'perfect' children, and that such processes serve only to further devalue people with mental and/or physical disabilities (see for example Davis 1987). The availability of genetic testing and counselling may help to sustain an image of a disabled child as a burden both to her parents and to society. Indeed, studies of the provision of amniocentesis lend some support to this concern (Farrant 1985). There is a danger that, rather than enabling parents to make decisions about their children's lives, genetic screening becomes an instrument of population control. Another question raised by the advance in genetics is whether resources for research and the development of screening procedures will become a substitute for providing support and facilities for people with disabilities and those who care for them. This is particularly worrying given the already existing low levels of financial backing for community provisions for people with learning difficulties. The development of genetic engineering raises fears of a new eugenics movement, which gives priority to improving the human or national gene pool over that of improving social conditions to enable people with learning difficulties (and their carers) to lead full and valued lives (see Stanworth 1987).

Finally, in cases of women with learning difficulties being sterilized without their direct consent, it is assumed that they must rely upon others to make decisions for them, and that they will be compliant with such decisions. In response to the 'Jeanette case' the Lothian Rights Group, a self-advocacy group of people with learning difficulties, pointed out that at no time had the views of self-advocacy groups been sought, even though the movement has been developing over the past ten years (Barry 1987: 5). Indeed, the perspective most missing in courts' decisions to sterilize is the voice of the individual herself, or of an independent advocate or group representing her interests.

Caring and dependency

> It's hard for ordinary women to go out, but they have husbands or boyfriends. Women with a handicap can't really go out (Atkinson and Williams 1990: 173).

Feminist social policy writers have drawn attention to the significant role women play in caring for others, either in an unpaid or paid capacity. Hilary Graham has summed up the experience of caring for women in general:

> [It] is the medium through which women are accepted into and feel they belong in the social world. It is the medium through

> which they gain admittance into both the private world of the home and the public world of labour market. It is through caring in an informal capacity – as mothers, wives, daughters, neighbours, friends – and through formal caring – as nurses, secretaries, cleaners, teachers, social workers – that women enter and occupy their place in society (Graham 1983: 30).

While recognizing that this experience varies for women according to their class and ethnic background, how far does it also apply to women with learning difficulties? Is it also for them the medium through which they gain acceptance into the public and the private sphere? We have already seen that one of these central caring roles – motherhood – is denied to the majority of women with learning difficulties. Yet it is still true that caring is an important aspect of the lives of many able-bodied women with learning difficulties. However, in their cases, it is caring as daughters and sisters, occasionally as wives, but rarely as mothers. Take the following example from a discussion of a group of women with learning difficulties:

> My mum died when I was small so now I look after my dad. I can't leave home because he needs me.
>
> Yes, my dad died. I cheer up my mum. She would be lost without me. I take her breakfast in bed.
>
> If your mum dies you need to stay at home to look after your dad. My dad likes me helping (Atkinson and Williams 1990: 175).

Such expectations of domestic labour and caring do not seem to provide admittance into the public world of paid work. Indeed, on the contrary, such expectations seem to lock women with learning difficulties more securely into the private world of the family or institution.

In the past 'mental deficiency colonies', hospitals and institutions benefited from the unpaid domestic labour of the more able female residents:

> In t' olden days I worked on a villa. Scrubbing on your hands and knees. I worked at night 'till 7.00 at night. Bathing them and putting them to bed, them being short-staffed. That's how they think I got me bad leg from, when I used to do a lot of scrubbing every morning and every night. They didn't have vacuums or things like that, like they have now. It was all kneeling, mucky, dirty side-rooms to do.

> We didn't get any money then. We'd not any money, we had to work for nothing. Work for nothing in them days. Then when it changed, you know the change over, they started giving them money and he said, 'you can buy some clothes now of your own!' (Atkinson and Williams 1990: 135).

It is not surprising to find that institutions were often reluctant to let their good female workers move back into or get paid work in the outside world.

Some women with learning difficulties clearly resent their restriction to the private sphere:

> My mum and dad don't let me go out unless I am on the centre transport or the Gateway bus.

> I make my own decisions but my Mum doesn't like me to go out. So if I go out I worry about her because she worries about me. It's boring being in every evening though (Atkinson and Williams 1990: 173).

These experiences suggest that while there have been attempts to create opportunities for independent living for people with learning difficulties in the community, these may well have different consequences for women and men. This suggestion is born out by a small research study carried out by Patricia Noonan Walsh in Ireland (Walsh 1988). Although there may be cultural differences in Ireland, her study nevertheless revealed two significant general observations. First, women with learning difficulties were more likely than men to live protected lives, whether at home, in a hostel or institution. Their lives followed a more restricted pattern of domestic duties and watching television rather than going out and engaging in social activities. Second, when women did go out, they were more likely to go to day centres and to travel there on a special minibus. Men, on the other hand, were encouraged to go to vocational centres where they could learn skills and learn to use public transport. In other words men had more opportunities to enjoy independent living than women.

In addition, Walsh found that the range of social skills taught to women and men reflected and reinforced this independence differential. Women were much more skilled at domestic duties – making the bed, setting a table, care of the kitchen. At the same time women were less able than the men at the sorts of skills required for personal care and independence – eating, drinking, table skills. While half the men in the study could shave themselves very few of the women were able to cope with menstrual care, although admittedly a more complex task. Such differences indicate the necessity of recognizing women's specific needs, and of creating the opportunities for particular skills to be acquired.

Experiences of racism

In their concern to protect women with learning difficulties from the outside world and, in particular, from sexual harassment and abuse, carers risk reinforcing their restricted and dependent lives. However, such fears for black women with learning difficulties may be compounded by the fear of racial harassment, as one young Asian woman with learning difficulties describes:

> In school I was bullied, sometimes called names like 'Pakki', but not in college. In a way I think I'm treated differently because I've a learning difficulty (Atkinson and Williams 1990: 91).

Discrimination in the provision of services may also restrict opportunities for black women with learning difficulties to develop new relationships and skills. For example, in 1984 a monitoring exercise was carried out in Harlesden by Harlesden Community Mental Handicap Team in the Borough of Brent, an area where 50 per cent of the population is black.[2] The team found that many black families with a member with learning difficulties were not using the services. This was not because they did not need the services, but because they did not know about the services, or more importantly, they did not perceive the services as being appropriate for them (Harlesden CMHT 1988). A similar study was undertaken in Lewisham by Contact-a-Family (CAF), a national voluntary organization which seeks to put families with children with disabilities or special needs in touch with one another. Here, too, it was found that black families were not using the service or involved in the organization because of its 'white image'. Alternatively, they were not being referred to the service by social workers, who assumed that since black people did not use the service, they did not require it.

A number of different processes contribute to the restriction of access and usage of services by black families. First, the services may be culturally inappropriate – for example, respite care, residential care or meals-on-wheels may fail to provide ethnic minority diets. Information about welfare benefits may be provided only in English; no interpreter may be available for a primary carer who does not speak English when assessments are being made, or when there are visits to hospital. Secondly, some practitioners may pride themselves on treating all clients the same 'regardless of colour, creed or class' – an apparent egalitarianism which may serve to obscure the specific needs of an individual black man or woman with learning difficulties. Although the acknowledgement of cultural differences is important, there may also be the risk of applying inappropriate cultural stereotypes. It may be assumed, for example, that extended Asian families with a member with learning difficulties can cope without outside support, or support may not be offered on the assumption that their families 'like to keep themselves to themselves'. Thus the failure of the service to provide opportunities for access may be attributed to assumed cultural idiosyncrasies. Racist and ethnocentric perceptions of black families may also result in negative assessments of parenting skills; parental concerns about inappropriate treatment of their children may be interpreted as being 'overprotective' or 'obstructive'. In Brent, concern with such practices led the mental handicap teams to examine the extent to which processes like 'normalization', assessment and portage were imbued with white cultural values, and assumptions of white cultural superiority.

In some situations racism may lead to a compounded form of oppression not only for the client but for the carer too. For example, in the study of black families' experiences in Lewisham, one mother of a child with special needs described feeling 'excluded' in her attempts to join in an all-white parents' self-help group. Ironically, such self-help groups are set up to protect parents, especially mothers, from the sense of isolation they already feel in having a disabled child. In this mother's case, this sense of isolation was doubled. (She was encouraged to set up an Afro-Caribbean parents' support group which was integrated into the local organization.)

The Harlesden experience suggested that while wanting independent living arrangements for their children, black families strongly expressed the desire to have these close to the family and within the neighbourhood. Black families were also more likely than white families to care for a member with learning difficulties at home. How far this is personal choice, dissatisfaction with existing services, lack of access to services, or a combination of all three, is not clear. However, it is clear that black women carers face additional problems because of their existing housing, employment and financial situation. Black families are more likely to live in flats and maisonettes, which makes mobility more difficult, and the mother's wage is likely to be a significant proportion of the family income – hence the loss of it is likely to be more acutely felt. In addition, black women are more likely to work in jobs which are physically tiring and have unsocial hours (Barrett and McIntosh 1985).

For all these reasons, it is important to develop strategies which counter the direct and indirect racism both within and outside service provision, and to incorporate them into anti-sexist strategies for people with learning difficulties. At the same time, strategies that begin to address these different issues have to be considered as part of strategies which seek to value people with learning difficulties, both women and men, and to give them a stronger voice.

Strategies for change

> When I told my mum I was in a women's group she said I was a girl. I said I was a woman. Now she knows I was right (Atkinson and Williams 1990: 173).

Strategies for improving the lives of women with learning difficulties have to do two things. They need to meet women's specific needs and ensure that general policies for people with learning difficulties do not discriminate against women. Specific needs that must be acknowledged are issues of menstruation, sexuality, sexual abuse, racial harassment, pregnancy, motherhood, the right to learn skills and get decently paid work, and to live independently where possible. The right to be considered as adult is general to all people with learning difficulties, but has specific meaning for women, as the quotation above illustrates.

In relation to sterilization, there is an urgent need for schemes and strategies which give greater recognition to the individual's own needs, experiences and opinions. The development of self-advocacy groups, advocacy schemes, support circles and shared action planning are all examples of strategies which seek to give greater recognition to the independent interests of individual people with learning difficulties, and to find ways in which these can be expressed.

There is also the question of developing alternative methods of sexual understanding and minimizing the risks of sexual vulnerability. Opportunities for people with learning difficulties to learn about and explore their own sexuality, as well as the consequences of sexual relationships, and of parenting, are still few and far between, especially for young women whose lives are limited to their home and the training centre. The stereotype of people with learning difficulties as childlike, having only a certain mental age, often makes it difficult for those who care for them to acknowledge or permit their sexuality. Sometimes, however, unconsented sterilization is approved to allow a woman the opportunity to develop a sexual relationship without risking pregnancy. The question here, however, is whether sterilization is being used as an expedient which avoids more time-consuming methods involving skilled communication, explanation and discussion (Craft and Craft 1978).

In some areas, workers in social education centres have helped set up women's groups for women with learning difficulties where such issues can be discussed. Such groups can encourage women to be more assertive and help counter stereotypes of women as passive, submissive and unable to make their own decisions. For example, in one group, women with learning difficulties discussed issues like going out after dark, self-assertiveness, relationships, and sex and Aids (Atkinson and Williams 1990). Through discussing, for example, the problem of sexual harassment, they began to understand their own vulnerability in a way which challenged the assumptions of passivity which often accompany the demand for women to be protected.[3]

The need to 'protect' vulnerable groups is often used to justify policies which ultimately have the effect of denying rights to those groups, through enforced institutionalization in the past and through sterilization without consent today. While the specific vulnerability of women with learning difficulties has to be acknowledged and tackled, this should be done in a way which increases their capacity to maintain their autonomy and assert their needs. Discussion in women's groups, advocacy or self-advocacy groups should focus upon the social conditions necessary to achieve these ends. There can be little case for the sterilization of a woman if there is any possibility that at any time in the future she may be able to understand her sexuality and be in a position either to give or refuse consent. Sterilization without consent can only be seen as a last resort, as a method of 'protection' which admits the lack of available means to enable the woman concerned to make an informed choice.

General strategies for people with learning difficulties should ensure that women are being treated equally. Sex education should not put the onus of understanding and responsibility for contraception entirely on the woman, nor the awareness of sexuality entirely upon the man. The movement for self-advocacy could ensure that women as well as men play leading roles in the running of groups. If appropriate, women's groups might operate alongside self-advocacy groups to ensure that women's needs are voiced. Social and work skills should be offered and taught equally to men and women, black and white.

The importance of involving clients, carers and the community in service planning is being increasingly acknowledged. In relation to black women and men, attention needs to be given to ways of involving black clients, parents, staff and people from black community projects and organizations in working parties which look at clients' or users' needs. This in itself suggests the need for local authority and voluntary services to develop links with the local black or minority ethnic community, and to involve representatives of local community groups, and particularly black or minority ethnic women's groups, in planning community care services and in developing, for example, translation services or advocacy services. In addition, workers may consider the possibility of setting up black carers' groups, or self-advocacy groups for black women with learning difficulties, as well as encouraging the organization of non-racist mixed groups.

At a more general level, the principle of normalization ought to be able to incorporate a critical awareness of the need to avoid replicating the gender and racial inequalities of the 'normal' world. The principle of normalization means that people with learning difficulties should be offered 'the same patterns of life and conditions of everyday living which are as close as possible to the regular circumstances and ways of life of society' (Nirje 1970). However, the concept of normalization carries the danger that, in so far as society is structured so that some groups or classes have greater power than others, then policy priorities will tend to reflect these power differentials. Thus the priorities established by service practitioners may reflect a white, male, middle-class view of the world.

Thus, in relation to women with learning difficulties, if we simply create the conditions and opportunities for women, for example, to marry, then this may well involve those women in a loss, as well as a gain in independence and status. They may feel more confident and valued in relation to the outside 'normal' world, but at the same time be entering a set of unequal personal relations in which they find themselves responsible for caring, cleaning, cooking and budgeting, or even subjected to violence and abuse. This is not to say that those who work with or care for women with learning difficulties should discourage marriage; it should exist as an option as it does for many people. But it does mean that discussions about gender inequalities, regarding, for example, the sexual division of labour, are as important a set of issues for young people with learning difficulties as they are for other young people.

As well as providing people with learning difficulties the opportunities to live like everybody else, we should also insist on their right to 'be different' and to be accepted as such. Some adults with learning difficulties live in small group homes; some people choose to live with a person of the same sex with whom they may have close and sometimes intimate relationships. In so far as these situations are the result of individuals' choice, then these should be encouraged and supported as much as aspirations to live an 'ordinary life'.

Finally, strategies to combat sexism and racism as they operate against women with learning difficulties have to be seen as just one aspect of strategies to combat structural, institutional and personal racism and sexism. At the level of institutional policy, therefore, the pursuit of equal opportunities policies in relation to the selection, recruitment, training and promotion of staff at all levels is an important part of the process of developing specific initiatives around gender and race and mental handicap. So, too, is the incorporation of issues of gender and race in training programmes for mental handicap workers in colleges, universities, local authorities and health authorities. More specifically, initiatives can include ethnic monitoring, not only of employees, but also of the provision and take-up of services, using action-research projects which look at access and user-perceptions of the service.

Such specific strategies aimed at the needs of women should not detract from strategies to enhance and empower people with learning difficulties in general. For practitioners these strategies involve critical awareness: of the service they are providing; of being sensitive to the needs of different users; of making services more accessible; of giving a voice to and empowering consumers. In so far as the issues of gender and race alert practitioners to the need for these processes of change, then they can also work to the general improvement of service provision for all people with learning difficulties and their families.

Acknowledgement

I would like to thank Mary Langan for her help in editing this article.

Notes

1 The situation of older women with learning difficulties is not dealt with here but many of the issues raised by Hughes and Mtezuka in this volume are relevant. In particular many older women are discharged into the community from institutions where they have spent their lives and they experience extreme loneliness.

2 Some of this information was gathered from interviews conducted by myself and Alison Tucker. In the process of preparing an Open University course 'Mental Handicap: Changing Perspectives' we interviewed Karen Salewski and Anna Dias of Brent Social Services, and Francis Fletcher and Miranda Parrot from Lewisham Contact-a-Family. My thanks go to them for these interviews and for access to reports prepared by them.

3 See for example the work of the Elfrieda Rathbone Centre in Islington in the video *Between Ourselves* from 20th Century Vixen (0273 692336).

References

Abbott, P. and Sapsford, R. (1987), *Community Care for Mentally Handicapped Children* (Milton Keynes: Open University Press).

Alexander, K., Hugarin, L. S. and Sigler, E. (1985), 'Effects of different living settings on the performance of mentally retarded individuals', *American Journal of Mental Deficiency* 9 (1), pp. 9–17.

Atkinson, D. and Williams, F. (1990), *'Know me as I am': An anthology of prose, poetry and art by people with learning difficulties* (Sevenoaks: Hodder and Stoughton).

Barrett, M. and McIntosh, M. (1985), 'Ethnocentricity and socialist feminist theory' *Feminist Review* 20, pp. 23–48.

Barry, N. (1987), 'The sterilisation debate: why weren't mentally handicapped people consulted?' *Social Work Today* 18 (37), p. 5.

Baxter, C. (1989), 'Parallels between the social role perception of people with learning difficulties and black and ethnic minority people' in Brechin and Walmsley 1989, pp. 237–46.

Blunden, R. (1980), *Individual Plans for Mentally Handicapped People: A Draft Procedural Guide* (Cardiff: Mental Handicap in Wales, Applied Research Unit).

Brechin, A. and Swain, J. (1987), *Changing Relationships: Shared Action Planning with People with Mental Handicap* (London: Harper and Row).

Brechin, A. and Walmsley, J. (eds) (1989), *Making Connections: Reflecting on the Lives and Experiences of People with Learning Difficulties* (Sevenoaks: Hodder and Stoughton).

Brown, H. and Craft, A. (1989), *Thinking the Unthinkable* (London: Family Planning Association).

Bryan, B., Dadzie, S. and Scafe, S. (1985), *The Heart of the Race: Black Women's Lives in Britain* (London: Virago).

Cawson, D. (1987), 'A case for castration, m' luds?' *The Health Service Journal* 26 March, p. 354.

City of Leeds (1932), *The Brochure of the Opening Ceremony of the Meanwood Park Colony Extensions* (Leeds: City of Leeds).

Connelly, N. (1988), *Care in the Multi Racial Community* (London: Policy Studies Institute).

Craft, M. and Craft, A. (1978), *Sex and the Mentally Handicapped: A Guide for Parents and Carers* (London: Routledge and Kegan Paul).

Crawley, B. (1988), *The Growing Voice: A Survey of Self Advocacy Groups in ATCs and Hospitalisation Great Britain* (London: CMH).

Davis, A. (1987), 'Women with disabilities: abortion and liberation', *Disability, Handicap and Society* 2, 3, pp. 275–84.

DHSS (1969), *Report of the Committee of Enquiry into Allegations of Ill-treatment of Patients and Other Irregularities at the Ely Hospital, Cardiff* Cmnd 3975 (London: HMSO).

Ehrenreich, B. and English, D. (1976), *Complaints and Disorders: the Sexual Politics of Sickness* (London: Readers and Writers Publishing Co-operative).

Farrant, W. (1985), 'Who's for Amniocentesis? The Politics of Pre-natural Screening', in H. Homans (ed.) (1985), *The Sexual Politics of Reproduction* (Aldershot: Gower).

Flynn, M. (1989), *Independent Living for Adults with Mental Handicap: A Place of My Own* (London: Cassell Educational).

Goffman, E. (1961), *Asylums* (New York: Doubleday).

Graham, H. (1983), 'Caring: a labour of love' in J. Finch and D. Groves (eds), *A Labour of Love: Women, Work and Caring* (London: Routledge and Kegan Paul).

Hall, S., Critcher, C., Jefferson, T., Clarke, J. and Roberts, B. (1978), *Policing and the Crisis: Mugging, the State and Law and Order* (London: Macmillan).

Harlesden CMHT (1988), *Mental Handicap in Multi Racial Britain: Whose Learning Difficulties?* Background Notes (unpublished).

McConkey, R. and McGinley, P. (eds) (1988), *Concepts and Controversies in Services for People with Mental Handicap* (Dublin: Woodlands Centre and St Michael's House).

Morris, P. (1969), *Put Away: A Sociological Study of Institutions for the Mentally Retarded* (London: Routledge and Kegan Paul).

National Institute on Mental Retardation (1980), *Sterilisation and Mental Handicap* (Ontario: NIMR).

Nirje, B. (1970), 'The normalisation principle – implications and comments', *British Journal of Subnormality* 16, pp. 62–70.

O'Brien, J. and Tyne, A. (1981), *The Principle of Normalisation: a Foundation for Effective Services* (London: CMH).

Open University (1986), *Mental Handicap: Patterns for Living* (Milton Keynes: Open University Press).

Open University (1990), *Mental Handicap: Changing Perspective* (Milton Keynes: Open University Press).

Potts, M. and Fido, R. (1990), *A Fit Person to be Removed* (Plymouth: Northcote House).

Ryan, J. (with Thomas, F.) (1987), *The Politics of Mental Handicap* (London: Free Association Books).

Shearer, A. (1986), *Building Community with People with Mental Handicaps, their Families and Friends* (London: CMH and King Edward's Hospital Fund).

Smith, H. and Brown, H. (1989), 'Whose community, whose care?' in Brechin and Walmsley 1989, pp. 229–36.

Stanworth, M. (ed.) (1987), *Reproductive Technologies: Gender, Motherhood and Medicine* (Cambridge: Polity Press).

Sumpton, R. (1988), 'Poverty and mental handicap', in S. Becker and S. MacPherson (eds) *Public Issues, Private Pain: Poverty, Social Work and Social Policy* (London: Social Services Insight) pp. 162–70.

Towell, D. (ed.) (1988), *An Ordinary Life in Practice: Developing Comprehensive Community-based Services for People with Learning Disabilities* (London: King's Fund Publishing Office).
Tyne, A, (1982), 'Community Care; and Mentally Handicapped People' in Walker 1982, pp. 141–58.

Walker, A. (ed.) (1982), *Community Care: the Family, the State and Social Policy* (Oxford: Basil Blackwell).
Walsh, P. Noonan (1988), 'Handicapped and female: two disabilities?' in R. McConkey and P. McGinley 1988.
Ward, L. (1988), 'Developing opportunities for an ordinary community life', in Towell 1988.
Wertheimer, A. (1981), 'Disability and income', in A. Walker and P. Townsend (eds), *Disability in Britain* (Oxford: Martin Robertson) pp. 156–74.
Williams, F. (1989), 'Mental handicap and oppression' in Brechin and Walmsley 1989, pp. 253–60.
Williams, P. and Schoultz, B. (1982), *We Can Speak for Ourselves: Self Advocacy for Mentally Handicapped People* (London: Souvenir Press).
Wolfensberger, W. (1972), *The Principle of Normalisation in Human Services* (Toronto: National Institute of Mental Retardation).
Wolfensberger, W. (1975), *The Origin and Nature of our Institutional Models* (New York: Human Policy Press).
Wolfensberger, W. (1983), 'Social role valorisation: a proposed new term for the principle of normalisation', *Mental Retardation*, December, pp. 234–9.

9 *Working with black single mothers: myths and reality*

Agnes Bryan

Introduction

Myths and stereotypes that negate the reality of the lives of black single mothers are pervasive in contemporary Britain. A social work practice that does not question these myths and reproduces negative stereotypes of black women is itself racist. White social workers need to understand the different and sometimes contradictory views held within the black community about motherhood and marriage, and how racism and sexism interact to shape black women's lives. This chapter critically assesses various models of social work intervention among black single mothers. It also surveys a black voluntary project to illustrate how an anti-racist and gender-sensitive approach can be developed.

It is important to acknowledge that the term black covers a great diversity of experience. It refers to people from different countries, races and cultures – from the Caribbean, Africa and Asian sub-continents – who are united by a common experience of colonial domination, immigration to Britain, and racial oppression. This chapter focuses on Afro-Caribbean women, who originate from Africa but whose recent ancestry is in the Caribbean. However, they are not a homogeneous group, and include people from many islands, some up to 1,500 miles apart, which have diverse cultural traditions. They, or their families of origin, may come from urban or rural areas. Also, the proximity of their experience of immigration varies: most Afro-Caribbeans in Britain today were born in Britain. Though they vary in socio-economic status, they share a common experience of racism.

Myths and reality

Myths and stereotypes about black women, and particularly black single mothers, are a reflection of racist perceptions of the black family and the relationships between black women and men. If the realities of black women's lives are to be understood, these myths have to be stripped away and replaced by an authentic understanding of their position in the context of post-war and contemporary racism. It is also necessary to understand the character of family relationships within the Caribbean, and the effects of slavery and colonization.

There is a widespread assumption that giving birth to illegitimate children is the norm for women of Afro-Caribbean origin. The black family is viewed as a disorganized unit, centred around a female–male relationship that is inherently unstable (Carby 1982). The young black woman is seen as sexually immoral and as uninterested in long-term relationships (Hooks 1982); the young black man is viewed as irresponsible, promiscuous and sexist (Staples 1982). The older black woman is personified as the matriarch who is independent but submissive, a child rearer, God-fearing and respectable; the older black man is considered to be weak, incapable of sustaining stable relationships, preferring a series of casual affairs. Rather than accept the role of husband and father, he is said to prefer cohabiting, living off the woman's income and refusing to support his children (Wallace 1979).

This mythical black family is seen to be 'populated' by illegitimate children reared by overburdened mothers, aunts and grandmothers (Staples 1982). The absentee or indifferent black father is blamed for reproducing the same pattern of male fecklessness. The overburdened mother forced to work full-time to support her family is accused of failing to discipline and control her children (Phoenix 1988).

Like all myths and stereotypes, these have some sort of distorted relation to reality – a reality that reflects the particular experiences of immigration and racial oppression which have had a profound influence on black women in Britain.

The first generation of Afro-Caribbean immigrants contained a high proportion of single men, cut off from ties of family, friendship and community. They were forced to find work and accommodation on the margins of society. From the beginning they faced hostility and racism. The women who were encouraged and chose to come to Britain to work, were seen as 'naturally suitable for the lowest paid most menial jobs' (Carby 1982: 219). Bridging the division between mothering and paid employment, they took on the roles of mothers, wives and workers simultaneously.

The state took little responsibility for supporting the black family in Britain during the immigration period, and ignored the needs of black women (Williams 1989). Instead, it promoted the notion of the black family as inherently pathological. Black women brought with them a value of 'non-dependence' (that is a non-reliance on the welfare state for help) in relation to child-rearing and family life. Coming from a Caribbean tradition of shared care and extended family networks, they found themselves isolated and lacking family support when they came to Britain (Carby 1982). Furthermore, their knowledge of, and access to, welfare provisions was limited. They did not look to the state for help, since discrimination in housing and employment did not instil confidence to ask for such help. The state made no attempt to provide services to meet the welfare needs of Afro-Caribbean immigrants and their families.

Although black women suffered isolation, loss of status and cultural devaluation, they attempted to reconstruct the female networks that provided support in the Caribbean context. They developed their own culture of resistance (Carby 1982).

Life has not been much easier for the next generation of Afro-Caribbean women who were born in Britain. Though their parents had experienced discrimination in employment and housing, in the prevailing conditions of economic expansion in the 1950s and 1960s most succeeded in establishing a livelihood for themselves and their families. By contrast, the economic climate of the 1970s and 1980s made it much more difficult for their children. The emergence of unemployment and mounting racial prejudice squeezed many Afro-Caribbean school leavers out of the job market, and undermined their prospects of setting up stable family networks.

Second-generation Afro-Caribbeans were less acquiescent than their parents to the racism of British society. Their outlook was that they had been born in Britain and were entitled to be treated equally as British citizens. Whereas their parents had been reluctant to accept welfare benefits, young blacks demanded them as a right. Young black women, often deprived of both a regular income and family support networks, insisted that the state should provide for their needs.

In the late 1980s, a more independent outlook emerged among a section of black women. Many professional working black women asserted their right to choose single parenthood, rejecting both dependency on the state and the conventional white family norm. However, they still experienced the general racial prejudice of British society and the inadequacy of public child care provision.

These developments have had major consequences for the relations between women and men in the black community, and for family life. For many young black men it has been difficult to play the role of male breadwinner in the conventional sense. They have been denied the chance to survive, even by hard work, like their parents, and are constantly abused by racist media and police harassment. They are very often forced to take on a hard macho image (Staples 1982). In a similar way, many black women have had to be strong and independent simply to survive, hold down a job and bring up children. It has often been easier for black women to get jobs in the service sector than for black men to break into spheres long protected by whites. The inevitable result has been greater tensions within the black community, between men frustrated by the denial of any opportunity to earn a living and self respect in society, and women forced to carry the dual burden of work and child-rearing on their own. On many occasions the black community has fought back against British racism, but the challenge has been contained by repression and integration.

An examination of the post-war experience of immigration and racism is important for any understanding of the experiences and position of black women in Britain. It is also crucial to understand the social value placed upon children, motherhood and marriage by black women, and how these values have been moulded by the effects of colonization and racism.

Marriage and motherhood

For black Afro-Caribbean women, motherhood and marriage are not inextricably linked. The high value placed on becoming a mother in the Afro-Caribbean community has a powerful influence on the attitudes and motivations of black women (Wallace 1979). White society's prevailing view of marriage as a contractual agreement entered into before children are conceived does not accord with the view of marriage held by many black women. White eurocentric assumptions preclude an understanding of why many black women become single mothers. These assumptions ignore the effects of structural racism upon the choices that black women (and men) make about their parenting relationships.

A historical perspective enables us to encounter some of the prevailing prejudices about the black community's attitude to marriage. Marriage in pre-colonial Africa was a contractual union which often involved long-lasting relationships, but it was not expected to be the all-encompassing, exclusive relationship of the Euro-American ideal (Sudarkasa 1981). Both women and men relied on the extended family and friends, as well as on their spouse, for emotionally gratifying relationships (Staples 1982).

Throughout slavery, and beyond, families were often divided, leaving women to head the household. Slave families were subject to disruption by the selling of children, fathers and mothers. The slave father lacked traditional authority over his family. He could not control the destinies of either his wife or his children. For the most part he could not provide for them or protect them. The role of patriarch was made virtually impossible for the black man during slavery and extremely difficult afterwards. However, despite these structural forces, some slave families were able to remain stable entities, thus demonstrating their power to survive the struggle against racism (Wallace 1979). Slaves were not usually required by their masters to form permanent unions, but many such unions did nevertheless exist (Gutman 1976). This suggests that blacks, both women and men, took traditional marriage and all it entailed quite seriously.

Afro-Caribbean immigrants to Britain continued the process of adaptation that had marked the evolution of the Afro-Caribbean family from slavery. Family patterns were influenced not only by White European norms but also by the standards and values that Afro-Caribbeans had brought from Africa and had adapted to conditions of slavery and colonialism. Respect, restraint, responsibility, and reciprocity were central values, and the common thread was commitment to the collective (Sudarkasa 1981).

As a result of these diverse processes of adaptation and change, a wide variety of mating patterns and unions exist among Afro-Caribbean families today, including legal marriage, common law unions and what are termed visiting relationships.[1] Many older couples have lived for years in common law unions until they have saved enough money to afford a wedding. For these couples, marriage is equated with improved socio-economic status. Many younger women, while having marriage as a long-term goal, are involved in some type of visiting relationship. More recently, however, some young women are questioning the institution of marriage and are choosing alternatives, such as single parenting (Ellis 1986). Young black women are more aware of sexism and of the sometimes oppressive character of marriage. Some women prefer for economic reasons to remain single, particularly if they are reliant on state benefits.

Given the fact that there is high unemployment among young black men and that they are more likely to be employed in poorly paid occupations (Staples 1986), it is not surprising that Afro-Caribbean women (who mostly marry Afro-Caribbean men) are not as likely to marry as white women (Phoenix 1988). Generally, however, the institution of marriage is still seen as the most desirable goal, and young black women are often pressured, both overtly and covertly, into marriage. Births outside marriage are not accepted as readily as white society tends to assume, and where a woman is a single parent a relationship with a particular man is considered important.

While many Afro-Caribbean women are ambivalent about marriage, they still place a high value on motherhood and child-rearing. Girls in the Caribbean grow up seeing older sisters 'mothering' younger siblings while their mothers work to support them. Bringing up children without the support of a man is not perceived by some black women as problematic. Any disadvantage attached to being a single mother is outweighed by the status given to motherhood.

From the days of slavery, women in the Caribbean have learned to adapt their family structures to suit their economic situation. Shared mothering released the birth mother to seek paid employment or make use of educational opportunities. Afro-Caribbean women of all classes, irrespective of marital status, accept responsibility for child care and child-rearing. Many women in the Caribbean who have had no children of their own care for and raise the children of others. Children may be cared for by grandmothers, aunts, or by close friends, godmothers and neighbours. The great importance attached to motherhood has provided women with considerable influence, authority and respect.

In Britain the difficulties black single mothers encounter are in part the product of structural racism. Today, the majority of Afro-Caribbean women of childbearing age are either British born or have lived most of their lives in Britain. They are, therefore, less likely to be influenced by historical patterns of behaviour in the Caribbean than by their daily experience of life in Britain (Phoenix 1988). Black single parents are often living on low incomes, have poor housing and limited access to adequate child care facilities. Moreover, the decline of the black extended family and shared mothering in Britain has further compounded these problems. Despite these difficulties, however, some young women may become pregnant and have a baby because they may see a brighter future with a child, which brings new meaning and responsibilities to their life.

In white British society a woman is expected to be emotionally and financially dependent upon a man, and any paid employment she does is seen as secondary to her primary role of being a mother (Calvert 1985). However, according to Hooks, black women have not had the 'opportunity to indulge in the parasitic dependence upon the male that is expected of females and encouraged in patriarchal society' (Hooks 1982: 82). Slavery forced many black women to be independent of black men and to struggle for their survival. Black women were not allowed to be passive. Within the Afro-Caribbean community in Britain and in the Caribbean, girls from an early age are taught strategies for survival. This creates a sense of independence, hence the image of the strong Afro-Caribbean woman who can cope with anything. At the same time, they are taught that it is desirable and indeed important to have a male partner. Thus female–male relationships are experienced in a contradictory way. On the one hand the belief is that 'getting married gives women added responsibilities, status and independence' (Ellis 1986: 8). On the other hand, men are seen to dominate women in an unequal power relationship.

Few black women have a choice about whether or not to go out to work, and this has enabled them to exhibit a certain spirit of independence, despite the fact that they are predominantly in low paid and low status jobs. However, they may still resent the fact that they do not have the choice to be supported by a man.

Black women's experiences as mothers and paid workers mean that they are often labelled as strong independent women, as matriarchs. White racism often identifies the black matriarch as the primary feature of the pathological Afro-Caribbean family (Hooks 1982). The black mother has nearly as much, or more, education than the black man; she works more frequently than the white woman; and her existence precludes the possibility of a strong black man, or any black man at all. Hence, black single mothers are seen as the product of this abnormal black family structure. We turn now to examine how these myths are perpetuated in sociological and psychological analyses of the black family, and in social work practice.

Social work and black single mothers

Black single mothers who become clients may be subject to different forms of social work intervention. These in turn will reflect the assumptions made about the nature and form of the Afro-Caribbean family, and the place of women within it.

An examination of the literature on the black Afro-Caribbean family reveals a number of distinct perspectives, including the pathological–pathogenic model and the adaptive–vitality model (Willie 1970; Staples 1978; McAdoo 1981). The first is based on the assumption that the black family is not only a dysfunctional and sick social unit, but produces sick and dysfunctional members of society. Thus, both black single mothers and their children will be viewed as problematic within this model. A social work practice which draws upon this perspective would focus its attention primarily on the individual black woman in isolation from her cultural and structural context.

But many problems – such as poverty, homelessness, unemployment and the effects of racism and sexism – are located, at least in part, outside the individual black mother who suffers them. This pathological–pathogenic perspective also overlooks how many problems are the product, not of the black mother's individual personality and behaviour, but of her inability to parent in a racist society in ways which she would ideally choose.

Denney (1983) further explains that the pathological–pathogenic model, which he calls the anthropological approach, assumes an ideology of assimilation and integration, thereby placing the responsibility for change on the individual black woman. It emphasizes a casework model which is largely therapeutic in nature, and gives the power to the social worker to decide who is suitable for social work intervention. Thus certain racial groupings may be defined as unsuitable for intervention, and black clients, such as single mothers, may be deemed unsuitable for social work help.

The adaptive–vitality model is based upon a different set of premises. It contends that adaptation by black people to socio-economic pressures and limitations should not be seen as pathological but as an indication of the strength and stability of the community. Karenga defines adaptive vitality as a people's ability to 'adjust structurally and ideologically in confrontation with society without losing its distinct character, to absorb stress and strain and bounce back with vigour' (Karenga 1982: 212). Thus the black family is viewed as a distinct institution with its own traditions and characteristics, not as a pathological variation of the Euro-American family. From this perspective, black women appear strong and independent, forming alliances and fashioning a way of life as mothers which enables them to resist racism, and adapt 'vitally' in the face of oppression. American writers like Nobles (1978), Staples (1978), and British writers like Ahmad (1988) and Dominelli (1988) explicate this view. They argue that the black family is unique, and thus so are the experiences of black single mothers.

The 'strength-of-the-family' model has been criticized for creating its own negatives while challenging the negatives of the pathological school. For example, Hill (1975) argues that one of the strengths of the black family is that there are strong kinship bonds which provide support for children and the elderly. This ignores the ways in which traditional extended family networks have been eroded in contemporary Britain, thus making it more difficult for black single mothers to combine paid employment with parenting. It also makes it easier for a racist society to abdicate its responsibility for black women and their families.

What is needed is an analysis which recognizes not only the strengths of black women and their adaptive vitality, but also understands the heavy burdens placed upon them which sometimes result in them being unable to cope.

In working with the black single mother the task is to encompass an appreciation of her specific culture, structural position, and her psychological needs. Given the difficulties this involves, there may be a tendency to focus too heavily on one of these facets of her life. For example, cultural explanations of her predicament need to be considered in the context of racism. Ahmed argues that there is a need to understand the 'dynamics and social forces which create a person's culture and frame of reference' (Ahmed 1986: 141). Over-reliance on cultural explanations runs the risk of ignoring, for example, the underlying emotional and psychological content of the black woman's problems. In work with young black single mothers cultural clashes between parent and child are often used as explanations for problems. But though parental conflict does arise as a result of conflict between traditional Afro-Caribbean values and Western values, this should form only part of the analysis. An analysis which takes account of cultural, structural, psychological and political factors is needed when working with black women.

Raising the consciousness of black women to bring about change is also crucial. White social workers may find it difficult to undertake this kind of work. Indeed, some black women may consider it an insult for a white person to explain to them their position in society, which is one of suffering racist abuse as part of their daily lives.

Therefore, it is self-evident that to be effective in giving support and help to black single mothers, social work practitioners need to raise their awareness of racism and examine their own attitudes towards black Afro-Caribbean women and their families. Furthermore, a gender-sensitive practice will be insufficient if it does not take account of the specific experiences of racism that black single mothers experience.

Working with black women: a voluntary project

The Family Support Service was a voluntary black self-help project which was set up in 1980. It was managed by black professionals with community participation. A black family worker from the local social services area office provided family work and groupwork. From the outset there was collaboration with social services, the housing department and the local health clinics. The women using the project for support, information and advice were mainly young black single mothers, all under thirty, either in late pregnancy or with new-born babies.

Most of the women using the project were dependent on the state in one way or another. This reflects Bruegel's discussion of the data which demonstrates that black single parents are less likely to be in paid employment and more dependent on social security than white single parents (Bruegel 1989). Racism in employment and the costs of child care mean that it makes less economic sense for black single mothers to take up paid employment.[2] The women using the project needed social security benefits but found themselves in an oppressive relationship with the state, which defined them as inadequate or as scroungers. This terminology is insulting to black women who are striving to be responsible parents, in circumstances characterized by poverty, deprivation and racism.

State provision for black women is of dubious value. Health and child care provision are inadequate, sometimes alientating and offered grudgingly. For young black mothers attending the Family Support Service, one of the greatest obstacles to finding employment, receiving education or training, was a lack of suitable day-care provision. Most of the women preferred to have their child in a day nursery rather than with a childminder because they believed the staff to be better qualified, and that as the majority of childminders were white they would be unable to provide an appropriate cultural experience for the child. Part of the hostility to childminders arose from the women's own feelings about a substitute mother who might question their adequacy as a young parent. However, statutory day nurseries are few, and the only guarantee of a place is if the child is 'at risk'. In the case of black single mothers there is an inherent contradiction. One the one hand they are seen as a high priority because, as a family type they are viewed as problematic, dysfunctional and unstable. On the other hand, they are denied nursery places because of racism in the system (Ahmed 1986).

The project had ambitious aims but scant resources. It was set up in the knowledge that the needs of black single mothers are dimly understood and that they are subject to negative and racist stereotypes. As black workers we believed that the women needed to remain at the centre of their communities, in order to receive the kind of support that would be beneficial to them as black single mothers likely to face isolation, unemployment, poverty, inadequate day care and possible homelessness and relationship difficulties. Our aim was to help and support these women, to develop confidence in their ability to manage the day-to-day running of their lives.

Work with individuals

During the early months of the project casework predominated. The casework relationship in social work has been criticized for locating the problem within the individual client rather than in the social structure. Yet casework need not ignore structural issues. Practitioners should recognize that sexism and racism are structural problems which have to be opposed by a variety of political strategies and tactics, as well as by working with the personal pain and feelings that the oppressive structures create. These feelings can be disabling and destructive.

Therefore we encouraged one-to-one casework, as well as working collectively. At an individual level, we empathized with their experiences as black women, whether or not we had children. Mindful of the power relations in the interactions, we tried not to be judgemental, and did not criticize them as mothers or carers. There was little concern about our statutory powers as only one worker was employed by the local authority. As we were all black women, they did not see us as traditional social workers and relations were easy and open. By helping the mothers to gain confidence and challenge their oppressive situations, whether within the family or the state, we helped to encourage a collective approach.

Our work did not fit within the traditional professional–client model. The women were not coming to be cured by the social worker. Our interventions were used as a means to explore the reasons for their difficulties and to reinforce positive feelings about their strengths. Their difficulties were understood within the context of racism and the problems involved in rearing young children in isolation. We were concerned with the mothers' subjective experiences rather than rehearsing the objective conditions of an oppressed group. Stress was placed on each mother's experience. We emphasized the importance of politicizing the personal, and recognizing the processes by which racism and sexism are internalized.

Groupwork

Most of the women participated in groups in which they could offer support to each other. The young mothers were encouraged to challenge society's prejudices and to appreciate the pervasive nature of racism from a personal and structural perspective. However, we were mindful of the fact that, while some women engage in and with groups, others find it intimidating and silencing. Hence, the value of one-to-one work was not underestimated or overlooked.

Groupwork provided the medium through which a number of wider activities, including a community childminding scheme and a sewing cooperative, were initiated. These activities generated collective support and helped some of the mothers to understand the need to take charge of their lives. They challenged the myth that black women only want to have children and be dependent on the state.

The childminding scheme alleviated the problem of isolation. Having children does not have to be constantly restrictive. The state sometimes puts too much emphasis on the care of children and not enough on women's needs. Women were given the freedom to have time for themselves, and the children were able to play with other children. They were accepted as the responsibility of the community. In the case of the sewing cooperative, the women made children's clothes, crafts, and rag dolls, and sold their products. Classes were organized with the aid of the local adult education institute to help educate the women about small business enterprise and running co-ops. This enabled the women to develop specific skills and to appreciate the possibilities of being both a mother and paid worker.

Other activities also enabled the women to take control of their lives. They organized short trips and longer holidays, raising the funds to pay for these activities, with some charitable support. Most of the planning and organization was undertaken by the women, with support from the workers. This provided a sense of collectivity and helped weaken individual dependency.

Consciousness-raising

Working with black single parents to understand the forces in society which act against them is a political activity. We encouraged the women to understand that their depressed and lonely life situations were the product of structural circumstances. This was not difficult. It flowed quite easily from discussions around relationships, both personal relationships with their men as well as relationships with various welfare agencies.

We supported women who, for one reason or another, did not receive the benefits they were entitled to, and who experienced humiliating interrogations by DSS fraud officers and appearances at appeals tribunals. We encouraged them to challenge the DSS benefit system. For example, we organized a campaign with help from the local Citizens' Advice Bureau around unclaimed benefits. The women gained experience in writing letters demanding their rights and in asserting their demands with people in power. Most importantly, they experienced a great sense of achievement and control over their lives.

Encouraging black women to see the politics of their situation and to take control is one of the most rewarding aspects of consciousness-raising. It was a crucial activity within the group. Women were encouraged to explore their experiences of being black women and to recognize their own value and potential to challenge things in their lives. They were helped to understand what change means and that the process is an ongoing dynamic one. It is the case that no one black woman's experience is more valid than any other, and that for each woman her experience is the truth.

Work with men

Our work with fathers and male partners was important in helping to challenge the notion of non-existent or irresponsible fathers. In fact, most of the women had some contact with their children's father. We were also mindful of the fact that the women saw the racism they faced as something their whole community experienced. Hence, we felt that it was essential to involve the men in some of the consciousness-raising activities and in the childminding scheme. Groupwork with men took place in single sex and sometimes mixed groups, and though at the beginning few wanted to be in an all-male group, this situation soon changed.

Discussions around female/male relationships proved to be rewarding for both groups. We emphasized four basic points. First, we insisted that black female–male relationships are no more problem-ridden or pathological than those of white or other ethnic groups. Second, it was important to recognize that real life unavoidably involves problems and problem-solving. That is, we cannot expect an unproblematic life but we can be resourceful in devising solutions. Third, it was important to recognize that not all black female–male relationships are in turmoil and trouble. However, there were enough relationships in difficulty to make discussion of the issues about black female–male relationships necessary. Finally, it was important to realize that any criticisms of the female–male relationship had to be seen in the context of living in white-dominated British society. Analyses of the major problems in black female–male relationships clearly revealed their social rather than purely individual nature. Therefore, to understand the negative aspects of these relationships, we had to understand the negative characteristics of the society which had shaped them.

Older women's support

One of the major features of the project was the role played by older women in helping to transmit traditional cultural values. This was made possible by working with the local black elderly project. Links were made via joint sessions with outside speakers on topical issues such as sickle cell anaemia, strokes and diabetes among Afro-Caribbean people. The older women also took part in the childminding scheme. Most of the discussions centred around generational and parental relationships, and once the trust and confidence had built up between the older and younger women, an informal network soon evolved. These women of different generations were able to discuss issues such as child-rearing practices, and to reflect upon the white view that Afro-Caribbean parents 'beat' and 'abuse' their children.

This informal care was supportive in many ways. It provided some experience of an extended family, in which such assistance is a family obligation. In such a family, members are not individuals in their own right so much as they are parts of a corporate whole.

Most of the women felt that the 'granny' figure was important and began to understand the strengths of the kinship network. The old women also enjoyed 'playing the granny', as it gave them the opportunity to maintain their dignity, and gave them a sense of worth by sharing their child care skills and their experiences of life in the Caribbean.

The assistance the older women provided may have been temporary, but regardless of duration the Caribbean-style woman-to-woman support helped break down the need for formal counselling or psychotherapy.

Resources for the black women

This project, set up for black women by black women became an invaluable resource. Welfare agencies were able to refer clients for help and support, and it served as a model for how to work non-oppressively and supportively with black single mothers.

We worked with the strengths of these black women, by drawing upon the values, survival skills and strategies of both the young and older generation. The idea of working with strengths is familiar to the black perspective. This concept is linked with the notion of ethnic pride and identity, aspirations of self-help and determination (Ahmad 1988). Group identity can be a great source of strength, and can sometimes provide a trusted informal support network, not just from friends, family members and neighbours, but from organizations. The Family Support Service was one such organization and, as a black organization, we were mindful that by using the strengths within the community we were not denying the need to gain equal access to social services provision.

Conclusion

This community social work project serves as one example of the type of activity social workers can engage in if they want to work in an anti-racist way with black women. Although it draws upon the experiences of black workers and highlights the importance of consciousness-raising, which may be problematic for white workers, it offers useful illustrative material for all practitioners.

White social workers need to recognize their social work practice as a political activity in which power operates at a number of different levels. They need to be aware of the power invested in them, by society, and the power relations between themselves and their black female clients. In addition, they need to understand other cultural patterns and traditions. A professional social worker should be interested in challenging the social structures in which the social work task occurs. This means understanding the racist context in which they find themselves. By taking account of racism, white workers can facilitate a better assessment of black single mothers. Instead of labelling them as inadequate mothers, white social workers should explore ways in which they can be more supportive and empower black women to make choices and take control of their lives.

Black women cannot be treated as if they were white in a colour-blind approach which negates their experiences as black women. A professional social worker is expected to empathize with the client, allowing her respect and dignity, and facilitating access to resources and expertise. A white social worker who accepts the black woman on a superficial level but does not attempt to understand her experience and her predicament is patronizing, and colluding with racism.

Notes

1 A visiting relationship can be defined as a 'semi-permanent relationship in which the man does not live in the same household as the woman but visits from time to time. The regularity and duration of such visits varies' (Ellis 1986: 7).

2 However, it is important to note that, overall, black women in Britain are more likely to be in the labour market, and less likely to work part-time, than white women (Bruegel 1989).

References

Ahmad, B. (1988), 'Turning the key to employment' *Social Work Today* 7, 20.

Ahmed, S., Cheetham, J. and Small, J. (eds) (1986), *Social Work with Black Children and their Families* (London: Batsford).

Bruegel, I. (1989), 'Sex and race in the labour market', *Feminist Review* 32, pp. 49–68.

Calvert, J. (1985), 'Motherhood', in E. Brook and A. Davis (eds), *Women, The Family and Social Work* (London: Tavistock).

Carby, H. (1982), 'White women listen! Black feminism and the boundaries of sisterhood', in Centre for Contemporary Cultural Studies, *The Empire Strikes Back: Race and Racism in 70s Britain* (London: Hutchinson).

Cheetham, J. (1972), *Social Work and Ethnicity* (London: Allen and Unwin).

Denney, D. (1983), 'Dominant perspectives in the literature relating to multi-racial social work', *British Journal of Social Work* 13.

Devore, W. and Schlesinger, E. (1987), *Ethnic Sensitive Social Work Practice* (London: Merrill).

Dominelli, D. (1979), 'The challenge to social work education', *Social Work Today* 25, 10.

Dominelli, L. (1988), *Anti-Racist Social Work* (London: Macmillan Education).

Ellis, E. (ed.) (1986), *Women of the Caribbean* (Kingston 5, Jamaica: Kingston Publishers).

Fulani, L. (ed.) (1987), *The Psychopathology of Everyday Racism and Sexism* (New York: Harrington Park Press).

Frazier, E. F. [1939] (1966), *The Negro Family in the United States* (Chicago: University of Chicago Press).

Gutman, H. (1976), *The Black Family in Slavery and Freedom* (New York: Random House).

Hill, R. (1975), *The Strength of Black Families* (New York: Emerson Hall).

Hooks, B. (1982), *Ain't I A Woman, Black Women and Feminism* (London: Pluto Press).

Karenga, M. (1982), *Introduction to Black Studies* (Los Angeles: Kawaida Publications).

Khan, V. S. and Ballard, R. (1979), *Minority Families in Britain* (London: Macmillan).

McAdoo, H. P. (ed.) (1981), *Black Families* (London: Sage).

Nobles, W. W. (1978), 'Aficianity: its role in Black families', in *The Black Family: Essays and Studies* (ed.) Robert Staples (Belmont, California: Woodstock Pub. Co. Inc.).

Nobles, W. W. (1981), 'African-American family life: an instrument of culture' in McAdoo 1981.

Phoenix, A. (1988), 'The Afro-Caribbean myth', *New Society*, March.

Staples, R. (ed.) (1978), *The Black Family: Essays and Studies* (Belmont, California: Woodstock Pub. Co. Inc.).

Staples, R. (1982), *The Black Masculinity: The Black Male's Role in American Society* (San Francisco: The Black Scholar Press).

Staples, R. (1986), *The Black Family* (Belmont, California: Wadsworth Publishing Company, Inc.).

Sudarkasa, N. (1981), 'Interpreting the African heritage in Afro-American family organisation', in McAdoo 1981.

Wallace, M. (1979), *Black Macho and the Myth of the Superwoman* (London: John Calder).
Williams, F. (1989), *Social Policy: A Critical Introduction* (London: Polity Press).
Willie, C. (1970), *The Family Life of Black People* (Columbus, Ohio: Charles Merrill).

10 *Women in residential work: dilemmas and ambiguities*

Cathy Aymer

Introduction

Residential care for children has increasingly become a residual service in which both workers and children may feel devalued and demoralized. Over the past decade social policy has made a priority of keeping children in their family of origin, or providing them with a substitute family through fostering or adoption. Residential homes have been maintained only as a last resort for children who cannot be sustained in either natural or substitute families. These are often adolescents with 'challenging' styles of behaviour, or other children with 'special needs'. As the overwhelming majority of child care workers, women are expected to play a range of contradictory roles in relation to children in their care. They are expected to act as surrogate mothers, nurturing and caring for children, and also, to act on behalf of society as 'father figures', as a source of discipline and authority over children defined as 'difficult'. Yet, as residential care has become a service of last resort, it has been starved of the resources required to provide the level of care necessary for the needs of the children involved.

A number of controversies have arisen in relation to residential care which highlight the contradictory pressures which particularly affect women care workers. There have been a series of sex scandals involving children's homes – where it has been alleged that male workers have sexually abused girls in their care, where adolescents in care are said to have been engaging in 'unrestrained' sexual activity, where lesbian and gay staff have been accused of 'molesting' children. Intense public concern over such cases, whipped up by prurient media coverage, has made women care workers more concerned to raise issues of sexuality in the context of residential care, while also making them more defensive about revealing their own sexual identities.

Another issue of particular concern is the disproportionate number of black children who have come into the residential sector since the 1970s. The implicit judgements that standards of child-rearing among black peope are in some way inferior, and that the black family is inherently pathological have become a focus of conflict between the black community and the social services establishment. The paradox that, though black mothers are judged inadequate in rearing children in the private sphere of the family, black care workers are allocated the task of raising these children in the public child care sector, is one that strikes black care workers with particular force. At the same time, black care workers may find themselves accused by the black community of complicity with the white social work system in removing black children from their families into contexts – through adoption, fostering or residential care – in which they may lose their ethnic and cultural identity.

This chapter explores the dilemmas facing care workers in the residential sector, focusing in particular on the contentious issues of gender, sexuality and race. Exploring these issues for women in residential work in no way denigrates the efforts of committed individuals, from whom I have learnt a great deal; by describing some of the complexities, however, I hope to illustrate why the job of residential social work often appears to present almost impossible difficulties.

Women's historical position in residential care

I began work in 1974 as an assistant housemother in a children's home in Yorkshire. The home was run on the model inaugurated by the 1946 Curtis Report on the care of children. Curtis-type family group homes were set up to give children in public care an experience as near as possible to 'normal' family life, by asking workers to become substitute parents. Typically, Curtis homes catered for eight to ten children of varying ages and both sexes, and were run by a married couple. Replicating the traditional family norm, the wife, designated the 'housemother', looked after the children and the household tasks, while her husband, the 'housefather' went out to work. The rest of the staff, often younger single women, were 'assistant housemothers'. For the children, the housefather was 'uncle', the female staff were all 'aunties'. In the home in Yorkshire, the housefather was a retired serviceman and he and his wife had already brought up their own family. 'Uncle' was clearly the boss, regarded by children and 'aunties' alike as the ultimate source of authority.

Whenever I described my job to anyone, the response was always a variation on two themes, either: 'You're wonderful, you must have the patience of a saint, I would never be able to do that'; or 'I don't suppose you need any qualifications to do that, after all it's what any good housewife would do?' Defining a professional role between Mother Teresa and Mrs Mopp is the difficult path that women in residential work are forced to tread.

In the early 1970s, residential work was demanding, poorly paid and characterized by long hours and irregular working patterns. It was the norm to work a split-shift system with no overtime pay or unsociable hours allowances. Family group homes reproduced the same sexual division of labour and power relationships between adult men and women and children as prevailed in the conventional nuclear family. Men represented authority and discipline while women performed personal care functions such as cooking, cleaning and laundry. Although the housefather sometimes undertook these tasks, this was seen as secondary and not his real job within the home. While the housefather could sit and watch television with the children, it was implicitly understood that the aunties could only justify their presence in the television room if they were doing ironing or mending. Work in the office and the allocation of money to children and staff were undertaken by the housefather. Liaising and negotiating with management and field social workers were also his responsibility.

In contrast, the housemother's tasks were restricted to child care and domestic functions. She would order the food and cleaning supplies, and take the children shopping for clothes. The aunties' contact with the outside world was mainly centred around taking the children to school, or on outings to the park, swimming pool or other forms of recreation. The children therefore experienced us as a hard-working group of women wearing 'pinnies' and doing 'women's work'.

In the late 1970s, however, there was a dramatic change in the pay and conditions of residential work. The introduction of the 45-hour week and paid sleeping-in allowances was followed by the 40-hour week with substantial increases in salary and the possibility of overtime payments. By 1979, workers in residential child care were able to benefit from a 39-hour week, and a reasonable salary and career structure. This change also came at a time when there was greater unionization of the workforce in the caring services. A small number of residential workers were members of NUPE, and others had begun to be recruited by NALGO.

The enhanced salaries and better working conditions meant that men began entering residential care in larger numbers. In 1977, 67 per cent of the staff working in children's homes were women and 33 per cent men (Howe 1986). My experience was that men were often to be found in the large observation and assessment centres. While some of the work was similar to that in group homes, the short-term and more specialist nature of assessment work meant that the professional role of the residential worker was more clearly defined. Men seemed attracted to this kind of residential work, where they were able to work closely with other professionals such as psychologists and psychiatrists, and thus their role was seen to have greater status.

Staff and children alike began to question the pseudo-familial relationships that were the legacy of Curtis. Staff were increasingly addressed by their first names and the terms auntie and houseparent began to disappear from the vocabulary of residential child care. There was a growing recognition of the social work task in residential work (CCETSW 1977), and staff were designated as care workers or residential social workers. The 'professionalization' of residential work meant that more men were working at the basic levels in 'ordinary' children's homes. Though men made up a smaller percentage of residential care staff, they accounted for a disproportionately large share of senior and managerial posts (Howe 1986).

Residential work began to attract more middle-class professional workers. Graduates and those who saw residential work as a career option or a means of gaining experience to enter professional social work training (and thereafter into fieldwork), came into residential work. This not only encouraged the professionalization trend but also had an impact on the sexual division of labour among residential workers. Smaller homes would now have cooks and other domestic staff, and a clear demarcation emerged between care staff and domestic staff. The latter were often older women recruited from the locality and paid substantially less than the care staff. Thus, while women in residential care were now recognized as performing social work tasks, it was still women who undertook the domestic labour.

Residential workers' tasks were more clearly defined as direct work with the children, and assessment of their physical and emotional development. This involved workers in much more contact with families, fieldworkers and other outside agencies. The office was no longer the domain of the housefather. It was the base for all workers in the home who were now perceived as a staff team.

However, although all residential workers were expected to do an equal job, in terms of care and control the sexual division of labour between men and women remained. The expectation that women would concern themselves more fully with the physical caring and emotional needs of children was taken for granted. Some men could use their physical size and presence as a means of discipline and control, while most women sought to find ways of negotiating control which were unrelated to their physical presence.

In the early 1980s child care policy shifted further away from institutional care to emphasize either supporting families in need or providing substitute families through fostering and adoption. Pressures to curb social services expenditure also encouraged the trend to close children's homes in favour of promoting cheaper community alternatives. Section 1 of the 1980 Child Care Act stressed the preventive function of social services departments in relation to children in need. In an attempt to minimize the phenomenon of 'drift' of children through residential care, departments also developed the notion of permanency planning, encouraging early decisions on long-term fostering and adoption in place of prolonged stays in children's homes (Thoburn, Murdoch and O'Brien 1986). This provides the philosophical base which now underpins policy and practice for social work with children and their families. A definite hierarchy has been established. First, the aim is to maintain children in their own homes or to return them to their families as soon as possible. Alternatively, substitute families should be found for as many children as possible, especially younger children. Finally, the dominant view is that residential care should be used only for those children and young people for whom the other alternatives are impossible.

A wisdom developed that regarded residential care as inherently bad for children, fuelled by scandals highlighting bad practice. But as Payne and Statham remind us:

> It is worth pointing out that some terrible things happen in families, often invisible and unknown to the outside world. Yet revelations of child abuse, granny bashing or marital violence are rarely used as arguments against the family. Rather the reverse, such evidence is used to argue the case for devoting more resources to strengthening, supporting and protecting the family (Payne and Statham 1988: x).

Social services departments had two objectives in recruiting substitute families. First it appeared to correspond to prevailing social work principles; second it enabled local authority managers to make savings on the costs of residential provision. The term substitute family came into use to replace the earlier term of foster mother. However, in assessing a family for its suitability as a substitute family, it is implicitly the ability of the mother to care for the child that is being assessed. Furthermore, since it is cheaper for a family to care for children rather than the state, foster mothers are being asked to perform their duties for lower pay than many state-employed professionals. More recently, foster parents, through the Foster Carers' Association, have demanded greater support from social services departments. They have requested more training and group support to help them to work with the more difficult children who are increasingly coming into their care.

Thus, residential care has increasingly become a residual service mainly for adolescents who are deemed to be at risk to themselves and others, or who have been emotionally damaged in their families. The impact of this reduction in service is that the task for women in residential work has become an impossible one, in that they must provide a service in which society has no faith. Thus the position is ambiguous. On the one hand they must provide a private function of caring which is highly valued, but on the other hand a public function which is demoralizing and devalued.

Sexuality in residential care: women's role

Sexuality is an underlying theme in all residential work. Although issues of sexuality often remain unspoken, they affect the work that residential workers, especially women, are asked to carry out. Sexual attitudes in residential care are no different from those found in the wider society, but residential work is an arena in which these attitudes are very graphically played out. Davis' work has been valuable in bringing the issue of sexuality out into the open and allowing us to recognize the importance of this aspect of residential work (Davis 1983). However, from a feminist perspective attitudes about sexuality can be fully confronted only if it is recognized that society implicitly expects residential staff, and in particular women, to control the sexuality of residents.

The adult world has grown up with myths about sex and sexuality, and these myths have led to certain assumptions about the types of adults that can be allowed to work with young people and vulnerable adults. Heterosexual women are seen to be able to care for both sexes, young and old, because it is assumed that the very act of caring renders them asexual (Ungerson 1983). The position of lesbians is slightly more ambiguous, for while they may be viewed as potential corrupters, their caring function may neutralize this concern. Consider also the myths surrounding a black woman's sexuality. These produce a tendency to categorize her as either the sexless 'mammy' or the sexual predator. The 'mammy' has a long history of being seen as suited to the role of caring. The sexual tigress derives her suitability from the assumption that she will confine her immorality to adult relationships.

In Curtis-type homes, the desirability of the presence of the husband as the father figure in the home contained an implicit assumption that his sexuality would be controlled by his wife. There have, however, been numerous allegations of heterosexual men abusing the girls in their care (the most recent example being the Greenwich Enquiry 1989) which have created unease about heterosexual men in residential child care. Adult women are expected to 'police' these wicked men, so that the ones who are perceived as safe can get on with their jobs. As well as protecting girls from predatory men, women are also expected to protect men from wicked girls who might seduce them or falsely accuse them of sexual misconduct.

Women care workers' role in 'protecting' their male colleagues from 'dangerous' girls has received little attention. Yet male workers commonly ask women to accompany them when they must deal with adolescent girls for fear of being sexually compromised. Women workers have complied with such requests because they have come to believe that this perception of risk is a reasonable definition of reality. However, even when women suffer sexual harassment from adolescent boys and adult males they are expected to tolerate them either as 'jokes' or as unavoidable hazards of the job. This appears to be simply another manifestation of how differently girls' sexuality is viewed from that of boys.

As in the larger society, girls' sexuality is placed under greater scrutiny than boys'. When women workers help to reinforce the stereotype of the predatory young woman, women workers miss the opportunity of establishing solidarity between themselves and young women. Thus their shared sexual vulnerability from adult males is denied.

The sexuality of black and white girls is also treated differently. In discussions about girls staying out late, uppermost in workers' minds is the fear that the girls may be in moral danger: this is translated into a fear about them becoming pregnant. While for white girls there is a strong impetus to protect them from becoming pregnant, it has been my experience that white workers do not see pregnancy for black girls as representing such a disaster. While it is true that black Afro-Caribbean families might more readily accept the child as part of the family, the initial impact is as devastating to the black family as to the white family. White workers misinterpret this acceptance of the child as meaning a lesser concern for the protection of the black girl's sexuality (see Agnes Bryan in this volume).

For black women in residential work, working with black girls places them in an ambiguous position. Black girls look towards them for clues of how to become adult black women, but if black women are still trying to find a way out of the tension between being the 'sexual predator' and the 'drudge', then they may portray an image to the girls that does not convey their confidence as adult women. Thus, black women may find themselves being dismissed as having nothing to offer black girls.

Caring for girls raises specific problems of sexuality for women care workers. The burden of asexuality that women workers carry means that girls may come to believe that sexuality equals dangerousness and may be forced to act this out. For if women workers have to be 'madonnas' the only available position left unoccupied for the girls is that of 'whore'. Girls who look towards women workers for examples of how to bcome adult sexual women who are not 'dangerous' may find little to help them. In families, young women and girls have the opportunity to gain some notion of their mothers as sexual beings. Their parents are likely to sleep in the same bed and they may experience babies being born into the household. Girls are denied this experience in residential care (although in Curtis-type homes children were able to see the housefather and housemother sharing the same room).

Furthermore, heterosexual male workers recognize that their own sexual feelings might be aroused by female residents and, in order to diminish their anxieties about this, project their feeling onto the girls. So, once again, in this interaction the girls are seen as dangerous while the men are deemed vulnerable. By policing the men, women workers inadvertently reinforce these prejudices. It is striking that when they have left care, girls often return with their babies, to show them off in a way which suggests that their newfound maternal status redeems their implied dangerous status, and so restores their reputation (Lees 1986).

Women workers, black and white, face difficulties in finding ways to respond sensitively and in an anti-sexist way to the emergent sexuality of young women and girls in residential care. The beginnings of mapping out what such a practice might look like will be discussed later.

Black women and substitute care

The early experiences of black women in Britain have been described by Bryan, Dadzie and Scafe (1985). In the 1950s and 1960s large numbers of black women entered the caring professions through nursing. However, it became clear that many had been directed to undertake SEN training, a lesser status qualification, with fewer opportunities, than an SRN. The disillusionment with this situation led some black women to move away from nursing and into residential work; initially with older people, but the beginning of the 1980s saw an increasing number of black women working with children.

At the same time many black children were being received into care and living in residential establishments (Ahmed *et al.* 1986). Much concern was expressed by black people about the over-representation of black children in care, particularly in some London boroughs. Much critical comment, however, failed to differentiate between boys and girls and thus ignored the specific factors resulting in black girls being taken into care. Research has been criticized for having 'failed to observe the differences and/or similarities in the situation of black boys and girls. Indeed there has been a total denial of the existence of black girls in the care system' (Barn 1990: 241).

Despite the fact that more black women were entering residential work, black girls and boys lived in residential establishments mainly staffed by white workers. The plight of these black children was discussed both in terms of their lack of appropriate physical care and their need for positive black role models. Many saw the solution to be to encourage more black carers into the residential child care sector.

This situation posed a dilemma for black women residential workers. Black people had begun to question the readiness with which white social workers intervened in black families and removed black children. They argued that social workers misrepresented black family structures as pathological because they did not fit the ideal typical nuclear family (Centre for Contemporary Cultural Studies 1982). Thus, while on the one hand children were being removed from black women who were deemed to be unfit to mother their children, black women as workers were seen as suitable substitute carers for these black children, and for white children. Hence, the black woman is expected to inhabit a public world of caring where her skills and knowledge are valued and a private world where these are questioned. As in relation to the specific issue of sexuality, this can create tensions and difficulties in the nature and form of relationship that is forged between the black woman worker and black girls in residential care. The shift away from residential care and towards substitute family placements has done little to ease the ambiguous position of black women.

The publication of a study of black children placed in white families (Gill and Jackson 1983) heralded one of the most important debates of the 1980s. Black professionals were able to make an impact on this debate (ABSWAAP 1983) by asserting that the development of a positive black identity is paramount in the decision to place a black child in a substitute family, and that same-race placement policies should be adopted by local authorities. Tizard and Phoenix (1989) have looked at the psychological arguments surrounding the opposition to transracial adoption and fostering, and reviewed the research in this area. They conclude that:

> One may or may not agree with the political objections to transracial adoption, and we would certainly argue that more

> black people should be encouraged and helped to come forward as adoptive and foster parents. But we would contend that the psychological objections to transracial adoption are not well-grounded in empirical data or theory. Differences are certain to be expected in the identity of black children growing up in white and black adoptive families, but there are not at present sufficient reasons to believe that the race of the adoptive parents should necessarily override other considerations in determining placement (Tizard and Phoenix 1989: 437).

These authors recognized that both political and psychological arguments have been used in support of the policy of same-race placements but they choose to discuss only the latter. By denuding the discussion of its political context, their conclusion becomes difficult to interpret. Why should black people be encouraged and helped to come forward as adoptive or foster parents if the 'other considerations in determining placement' can successfully be met by white substitute families? Are we also to assume that these 'other considerations' are ones that have been well-grounded in empirical data and theory?

Hidden within this debate is the issue of mothers and mothering. Gill and Jackson indicate that in the families they studied, it was the mothers who were the primary carers (Gill and Jackson 1983: 23). Hence, the object of study was one in which black children were moved from black mothers to white mothers, sometimes via the care of black and white women in residential care. This may shed some light on some of the angry feelings that are aroused by this issue. It appears that white mothering is seen as preferable to black mothering.

Furthermore, it appears that black mothering, whether in private homes or in residential establishments, is regarded as inferior to white mothering. Thus, the particular qualities of black mothers in assisting the development of the identity of black children are not recognized. The issues surrounding the identity of the black girl placed in a white family are no different from those that we have discussed for the girl in residential care. How does she get clues from her white mother of how to become an adult black woman?

In late 1989 Croydon social services department headlined the case of an infant who had been placed temporarily with a white family while a black family was sought as a permanent placement. A lengthier process than had been anticipated resulted in the child spending the first year of its life with the white foster-mother, who became increasingly attached to the child and applied for permanent custody as an adoptive parent. When this was refused, in line with council policy that black children should go for long-term fostering and adoption to black families, the foster mother sought to make the child a ward of court, to prevent its removal from her care.

In response to intense public discussion around the issue the social services minister intervened to direct placement agencies to reconsider the policy of same-race placements. This unprecedented intervention by a government minister in a professional decision suggests that there is a question to be asked about the relative power of black mothers and white mothers. Do white women who feel 'deprived' of their ability to mother have greater access to power than black women who may feel similarly 'deprived'?

The first avenue of power is the 'power of theory'. Here we have two theories: attachment versus racial identity. They compete for credibility. Respectability is given to attachment theories (propounded by white professionals) as opposed to racial identity theories (propounded by black professionals). The second avenue of power is that of the structure which has the power to decide what is in the best interests of the child. The two avenues are obviously connected, in that decision-makers either explicitly or implicitly draw on these theories in order to justify their decision.

This discussion about the issues surrounding the placement of black children in care, whether it is in a residential home or substitute placement, throws into sharp focus the ambiguous and difficult position of black women as both residential workers and substitute carers. What black women workers share with 'natural' black mothers is a set of experiences which represent a denial of the specific contribution they can make to a black child's upbringing. As a result, they are constantly having to confront the racist structures which impede this process. It is to some of these issues that we now turn.

Race, gender and sexual identities

Recently, writers have considered the development of anti-racist and anti-sexist practice in social work (for example Ahmed, Cheetham and Small 1986; Dominelli 1988; Dominelli and McLeod 1988). Their analyses and strategies are applicable to the residential situation. In addition, however, residential workers must develop a practice that is sensitive to understanding the emotional development of young people.

Although much emphasis is placed on physical care, the fundamental task in residential work is assisting young people with their development of a complex set of identities and helping them to understand the interplay between them. The residential worker then acts as a facilitator through whom young people can begin to make sense of themselves and the world in which they live.

For society, what is normal is defined as male, white, heterosexual, able-bodied, financially secure, and so on. Children in residential care are aware that their in-care status defines them as 'deviant', either by virtue of not living in a family or by real or imagined offending behaviour. They recognize also that they often differ from the norm in at least one other characteristic, and for most in several important respects.

The question for women workers is how to be an authentic person with a complex set of identities (not the ones described by society as normal and good) when the process of residential work limits this authenticity. When working with girls, women often hear the challenge: 'You're not my mother, you can't tell me what to do.' Young women have a notion of what mothers are and that they have some rights to discipline and make rules for their daughters. Women care workers cannot pretend to be mothers of girls in care, but neither can they deny the authority that is ascribed to them as social workers employed by the state. If women workers are to become real role models for girls in residential care, this means that part of the residential task is the disclosure of themselves as black and white sexual women.

What does disclosure of sexuality mean? It means creating a culture in which sexuality is no longer secret and everyone feels free to be open about their own sexuality. Women care workers should challenge the myth that they are asexual, and staff groups should openly discuss issues of sexuality and sexual identities. Adequate time should be set aside for these discussions. A dialogue should be opened up between women workers and between male and female workers, so that men can also acknowledge their sexual feelings in order not to project these onto the girls in their care. Workers should explore the myths surrounding dangerousness and vulnerability.

This openness should be extended to discussions of sexuality and sexual identities with young people. Often adults limit this discussion to sex education, which is defined as the giving of contraceptive advice. This is clearly important, but there should also be a recognition that sexuality is about feelings about self and others, body image, behaviour and lifestyles. Such openness about sexuality would lead to proper dialogue between women workers and girls, enabling them to discuss their shared concerns.

In relation to race, disclosure would mean that workers openly recognize their differences and the meanings attached to these differences. This would enable workers to determine whether stereotypical views of themselves and each other are being portrayed and allow commonalities to be explored. It would allow young people to deal with uncertainties and anxieties surrounding their own process of becoming adults who have to confront a complex set of racial and cultural realities. Workers would be able to determine how to form alliances in order to develop strategies for fighting racism within the residential setting. A clear example can then be given to young people to assist them in dealing with issues of race and racism, so that the notion of racial identity can be explored with sensitivity and safety.

Discussions around gender suggest that taken-for-granted assumptions of what it means to be a woman or man must be open for debate within the residential establishment. In particular, consideration needs to be given to the ways in which roles and expectations are socially constructed and to the impact of the sexual division of labour on people's lives. For girls it is important that they enter into discussion with women about how roles can be internalized in a way which limits the aspirations of girls leaving care.

Conclusion

Though residential care for children is a declining sector, it is certain to remain 'home' for a significant number of children who will have to overcome major disadvantages in the process of becoming adults capable of participating freely and equally in society. It will also remain 'work' for many poorly paid, highly dedicated and predominantly female care staff. This is why it is so important that the issues of gender, race and sexuality discussed here are taken up by residential workers, social work educators and policy-makers. If the residential experience is to become a positive one for children and young people, and for care workers too, these issues must be confronted.

Indeed if these problems are openly acknowledged and tackled, the group living situation of the progressive children's home may provide a positive alternative to the conventional nuclear family, instead of being regarded as a poor substitute. A home in which male and female care workers and young people are able to explore their identities together may provide young people with a much greater awareness of the complexities of gender, race and sexuality than the private world of the conventional white nuclear family, with its oppressive patriarchy and secretive sexuality.

In recent years there has been much discussion of the need to equip young people leaving residential care with the requisite social skills to survive outside the security of the home. The approach to the problems of 'independent living' has been characteristically gendered and narrow. Thus, young women are particularly expected to acquire practical domestic skills, while this is a lower priority for boys, who in turn are expected to find somebody of the opposite sex as rapidly as possible to perform such functions. Yet, though both young women and boys leaving residential care face considerable practical difficulties in finding work, decent housing and organizing their lives, they also face emotional, psychological and social problems.

The basic requirement for independent living is a coherent sense of self. This means a sense of individual identity and self-confidence which can provide the emotional resources necessary to withstand adversity. The fundamental task of residential care workers is to promote this sense of identity, to overcome their own sense of what Goffman characterized as 'spoiled identities' (Goffman 1963). Helping young people to overcome these problems means empowering them, enabling young people who may be black, female, poor, disabled, or in any way deviant from the socially prescribed norm, to cope in a hostile world.

To empower young people in care is undoubtedly a more difficult task than to teach them how to cook, shop, budget, wash clothes and perform all the other practical tasks of day-to-day survival. It is a greater challenge to care workers because it confronts them with their own, perhaps unresolved, problems of identity and allegiance. But if residential care is to become something more than a dump for a new residuum of problem children and a ghetto of frustrated professionals, then the strategies of anti-discriminatory social work offer the only way forward.

References

Ahmed, S., Cheetham, J. and Small, J. (1986), *Social Work with Black Children and their Families* (London: Batsford).

Association of Black Social Workers and Allied Professions (1983), *Black Children in Care* Evidence to House of Commons Social Services Committee.

Barn, R. (1990), 'Black children in local authority care: admission patterns', *New Community* 16 (2), pp. 229–46.

Bryan, B., Dadzie, S. and Scafe, S. (1985), *The Heart of the Race* (London: Virago).

CCETSW (1977), *Residential Work is Social Work* (London: CCETSW).

Centre for Contemporary Cultural Studies (1982), *The Empire Strikes Back* (London: Hutchinson).

Davis, L. (1983), *Sex and the Social Worker* (London: Heinemann).

Dominelli, L. (1988), *Anti-Racist Social Work* (London: Macmillan).

Dominelli, L. and McLeod, E. (1988), *Feminist Social Work* (London: Macmillan Education).

Gill, O. and Jackson, B. (1983), *Adoption and Race* (London: Batsford).
Goffman, E. (1963), *Stigma: Notes on the Management of Spoiled Identity* (Englewood Cliffs: Prentice Hall).

Howe, D. (1986), 'The segregation of women and their work in the personal social services', *Critical Social Policy* 15, pp. 21–35.

Lees, S. (1986), *Losing Out: Sexuality and Adolescent Girls* (London: Hutchinson).

Payne, C. and Statham, D. (1988), 'Residential services are a social need', *Community Care*, 24 November.

Thoburn, J., Murdoch, A. and O'Brien, A. (1986), *Permanence in Child Care* (Oxford: Basil Blackwell).
Tizard, B. and Phoenix, A. (1989), 'Black identity and transracial adoption', *New Community* 15 (3), pp. 427–37.

Ungerson, C. (1983), 'Women and caring: skills, tasks and taboos', in E. Gamarnikow *et al.* (eds), *The Public and the Private* (London: Heinemann).

11 *Lesbians, the state and social work practice*

Helen Cosis Brown

Introduction

As a result of a decade of campaigning by various pressure groups, around issues of equal opportunities, the Central Council for Education and Training in Social Work (CCETSW) now insists that candidates for the Diploma in Social Work (DipSW) must demonstrate their competence in non-discriminatory and non-oppressive social work practice (CCETSW, 1989). Despite the fact that lesbians are discriminated against in society, and in traditional social work practice, they have often been ignored in progressive developments in social work. It is therefore of some urgency that practitioners, managers, students and teachers become more aware of the oppression of lesbians and how it can be combated.

Lesbians do not constitute *per se*, a social work client group but lesbianism, as an issue, often arises in the social work context. There have been a number of child custody cases in which the mother's lesbianism has been deemed damaging to her child's development (Radford and Cobley 1987). There have been recurring controversies over the refusal of local authorities to recognize lesbians as suitable for fostering and adoption. Lesbianism has sometimes become an issue for social workers themselves, when lesbian residential and child care workers have been sacked on the grounds that they are a danger to children (Davis 1983: 60).

In practice, social work agencies tend to deal with lesbians in one of two ways. Either the woman's specific needs as a lesbian remain unrecognized and ignored, or her lesbianism becomes the central preoccupation, the prism through which her every word and action is interpreted. The first reaction is particularly common in relation to older lesbians, whose needs with respect to bereavement or institutional care may, as a result, be neglected. The second is the characteristic response to younger lesbians, in particular those who are explicit about their sexual identity. Both approaches are the result of the influence of prejudices and stereotypes which lead to a failure to consider the unique situation and needs of every individual.

Effective social work with lesbians must begin from a rejection of prejudices and stereotypes and a recognition of the individuality of every person. To offer a non-discriminatory service to a lesbian it is necessary to understand not only the general character of her oppression, but also to appreciate how she experiences oppression in her particular situation.

This chapter begins with a survey of the state of social work theory in relation to lesbianism. At a time of unprecedented flux in social work theory in general, there is considerable scope to push the issue of lesbianism higher up the agenda, to encourage a higher standard of discussion about current trends and policy developments. The second theme is the impact on lesbians of local government initiatives, both the progressive activities of a few Labour councils, and the more backward outlook of others, particularly in the homophobic climate encouraged by section 28 of the 1988 Local Government Act. The third theme is the issue of 'coming out' for lesbian social workers. The chapter concludes by looking at two areas of social work practice with important implications for lesbians – work with older women and child protection – and raises some ideas for the future of social work policy and practice.

Social work theory and lesbianism

Social work theory in relation to homosexuality has drawn from sociology, psychology and psychoanalytic theory. Much of this tradition regards homosexuality as a pathological deviation for which some *cause* must be found, hence the preoccupation with genetic theories, the influence of early social learning experiences, theories of heterophobia and seduction, and social interaction models (Hart and Richardson 1981). In most discussions about male and female homosexuality, sexual behaviour is seen to be the defining characteristic of identity. Reality, not surprisingly, is more complex. The question of defining oneself as a lesbian or being defined as a lesbian is an ongoing series of difficult processes, which will be different for different women. Many women experience sexual relationships with women, but would never perceive of themselves as lesbians. Some women would refer to having 'gay relationships' but not to adopt a total identity as a lesbian. Some black women may not identify as lesbians in certain situations, making a rational choice about not wanting to take on racism and homophobia at the same time in a given situation (Carmen, Gail, Shaila and Pratibha 1984; GLC 1986a; Parmar 1989).

Because lesbianism is pathologized, and lesbians are an oppressed group, lesbian identity cannot be reduced to the involvement of individuals in particular sexual acts; lesbianism is *socially* constructed:

> The process whereby a woman identifies as lesbian or not, and (if she does) the meaning and significance such an identification will have for her, will be influenced by the wide social meaning ascribed to lesbianism that she encounters, as well as the specific responses of significant others to this information (Richardson 1981).

Social work theory is still heavily imbued with the psychoanalytic notions integrated into its body of knowledge in the late 1940s and 1950s (Yelloly 1980; Pearson *et al.* 1988). Social work's adaptation of psychoanalytic thinking and psychodynamic principles was often simplistic, reinforcing conventional prejudices about masculinity, femininity, correct gender-identification and heterosexuality (Wilson 1977). Although social work theory has gone through many metamorphoses since the 1950s, much of its theory of gender and sexuality has remained intact, continuing to reflect 'common sense' public opinion.

Academic psychology has had difficulty in accepting lesbianism as anything other than pathological (Hart and Richardson 1981; Kitzinger 1987). Lesbianism has been theorized as an arrested state, a wish to be male, a denial of femininity, a measure of an individual's immaturity. The common theme of these diverse interpretations is that the lesbian is sick. However, during the 1960s, the pathologizing model was challenged by the liberal-humanist approach, which affirmed the value of the individual and the importance of facilitating each individual's 'self-actualization'. The liberal-humanists have been criticized for depoliticizing lesbianism (Kitzinger 1987: 45), though from the perspective of social work, this seems an unfair judgement on an approach which at least freed lesbians from the label of mental illness.

In the field of sociology, in the 1960s and 1970s symbolic interactionists examined how homosexuality was constructed and studied the consequences for the individual of labelling sexual deviance (Gagnon and Simon 1973; Plummer 1975). The symbolic interactionists were concerned 'with sexual meaning and the way it is socially constructed and socially patterned' (Plummer 1975: 222). However most of this work was narrowly focused on male homosexuality; lesbianism tended to be simply 'tacked on', often inappropriately.

The central theme of the more progressive psychology and sociology of the 1960s and early 1970s was that whether we were lesbians, gay men or heterosexuals, we were all the same underneath. 'Generally, then, the task of liberal social science with regard to lesbians has been one of normalization through humanization, with a touch of feminization thrown in for good luck' (Faraday 1981: 126). These theoretical influences encouraged social work's emphasis on individual casework. There was little recognition of the political issues involved in the oppression of homosexuality, or of the potential of collective resistance.

The 'radical social work' tradition of the 1970s viewed the casework model as excessively individualistic and influenced by pathological theories about the working class. However, radical social work has itself often been criticized for neglecting the specific experiences of women and black people; issues of homosexuality also remained marginal to its concerns.

One of the interesting developments of the 1980s was the emergence of feminist therapy out of the psychodynamic tradition. Lesbians and gay men have found psychodynamic approaches useful in setting up counselling services, and psychotherapeutic thinking has proved fruitful in developing a deeper awareness about lesbianism (Ryan 1983; Boston Lesbian Psychologies Collective 1987; Trevithick and Ryan 1988). In using psychodynamic theory to understand how the processes of internalization and identification with oppression take place, lesbians and gay men have followed the pioneering studies of parallel processes in the experience of racial oppression (Fanon 1967).

Recent feminist social work literature has had little, beyond generalities, to say about lesbians (Brook and Davis 1985; Dale and Foster 1986; Hanmer and Statham 1988). There is little appreciation that lesbians are as diverse as heterosexual women, the only commonality being their oppression as lesbians. How individual women respond to and cope with that oppression will also be dictated by their own individual life histories and individual psyches, their relationship to their families, their relationship to their cultures, whether they are black or white, middle-class or working-class, Jewish or gentile, able-bodied or living with a disability. Generalizations about lesbians are useful in social work only as tentative questions to be used in trying to understand a particular individual.

Although Dominelli and McLeod only briefly touch on lesbianism, they do recognize the diversities and complexities among lesbians (Dominelli and McLeod 1989). However, in presenting a positive perspective on lesbianism, they end up with a rather romanticized view of reality:

> For feminists, lesbianism is no longer lodged in the realms of the psychopathological and has been increasingly recognised and

> legitimated as an intensely expressive form of relationship in its own right by substantial numbers of women within the women's movement (Dominelli and McLeod 1989: 88).

Unlike Dominelli and McLeod, many social work academics and writers still regard lesbianism as a pathological condition. Even at the liberal end of the continuum there is still a preoccupation with causation. Some writing demonstrates sheer ignorance about lesbians. Take this example from a recent book on sexuality in social work:

> The homosexual social worker may experience difficulty in understanding heterosexual problems, particularly in relation to family planning and the stresses that contraception can place upon a sexual relationship (Christopher 1980: 278).

This author appears to be unaware of the fact that most social workers are women (Howe 1986), and that most lesbians have had experience of heterosexual relationships (Wolff 1971). Would the same comment be made in relation to lesbians' need to be understood in terms of their sexual practice by heterosexual social workers? The same author goes out of her way to help the heterosexual social worker with this very problem by detailing what lesbians are supposed to do in bed. However, despite its weaknesses, this book has the merit of being one of the few social work publications that tries to address why heterosexuals are so obsessed and anxious about homosexuality. *Sex and the Social Worker* is another mainstream publication which adopts a more sophisticated handling of the issues, and gives a sensitive account of social work intervention (Davis 1983).

It is easy to criticize the liberal-humanist position to lesbianism as being too individualistic. However, a more politicized approach, which has an understanding of collective oppression but loses sight of the individual, can be equally oppressive. Within social work we need to integrate the strengths of both perspectives.

To equip social workers with the knowledge and skills necessary to offer an adequate service to lesbian clients is a difficult task. As lesbians find themselves in a defensive position, in relation to their lives and rights, much writing relevant to social work is arguing for an anti-discriminatory social work response. While, given current trends, this is essential, it does not resolve more complex debates around lesbian psychologies, lesbian parenting, lesbian mental health issues, lesbians and the ageing process, and so on. Some more exploratory work is being done in the United States, looking in a more complex way at lesbian psychology and the impact of oppression in a non-pathologizing way (Boston Lesbian Psychologies Collective 1987). Similar work needs to be undertaken in Britain, for social workers to begin to offer a sensitive and appropriate service to lesbian clients.

Local Authorities – the 1980s into the 1990s; a move from oppression to liberal acceptance?

The 1980s saw Labour-controlled authorities in London and other cities beginning to examine what equal opportunities, in relation to sexual orientation, might entail. Three separate movements have affected local authorities' policies in relation to lesbians and gay men. First, within the Labour Party there has been the demand for autonomous organization of different groups (women, gay men and lesbians, and black people). Although these demands have faced much resistance, they have had some impact (Tobin 1990). In 1985 the TUC and the Labour Party Conference for the first time passed resolutions supporting lesbian and gay rights (Labour Campaign for Lesbian and Gay Rights 1986). Second, the Greater London Council (GLC), under Ken Livingstone, gave a lead in raising lesbian and gay issues and encouraged other local councils to follow. In its last years the GLC produced some important publications which had some influence on the position of workers within local authorities and local authority services (GLC and the GLC Gay Working Party 1985; GLC 1986a; GLC 1986b). The GLC's *London Charter for Gay and Lesbian Rights* (GLC and the GLC Gay Working Party 1985) examined social services provision, and the changes necessary for it to begin to provide an appropriate service for lesbians and gay men. Other local authorities tried to become more receptive and accountable to the public and more open to the demands of campaigning groups. For example, one London local authority involved the Lesbian Custody Group, a women's centre, the Nalgo Lesbian and Gay Group and the local law centre in meetings with the social services directorate, which would previously have been inconceivable. Whether the benefits of these initiatives filter through to lesbian workers and clients is more difficult to assess.

The third movement was the development of a strong lesbian and gay lobby within the National And Local Government Officers Association (NALGO). Changes in the area of equal opportunities within local authorities have come about as a result of a complex process of interaction between NALGO, the National Union of Public Employees (NUPE), black workers' groups, and management. As within the Labour Party, black workers and lesbians and gay men have faced considerable resistance to their struggle for autonomous organization since the early 1970s (McKay 1984). Much of the early activity took place around supporting workers who had been sacked from residential social work jobs on the grounds of being lesbians or gay men. In the mid-1970s, NALGO's national conference resolved to include 'sexual orientation' into equal opportunities agreements. By 1983 the pressure of lesbians and gay men within NALGO had led to the establishment of annual national NALGO lesbian and gay conferences. The NALGO lesbian and gay group has always campaigned simultaneously around workers' rights and appropriate service provision for the lesbian and gay public. Discussions of service provision covered a wide range, including a lesbian and gay parenting conference in 1986. In 1987, the NALGO Conference accepted a motion submitted to adopt the Lesbian Mothers' Custody Charter, to end discrimination against lesbian mothers. This was an important achievement, given that many social workers are NALGO members, and may be involved in custody cases. The pressure exerted by NALGO both nationally and locally on employers has undoubtedly had some impact on the development of policy and practice reviews of services to the lesbian and gay public. It has certainly contributed to the inclusion of sexual orientation in local authority equal opportunities policies. In response some local authorities (e.g. Haringay, Camden) set up lesbian and gay units to monitor provisions for lesbians and gay men. Others have used their existing lesbian and gay workforce to help review services.

These three movements had considerable impact on lesbian social workers and residential workers, day care workers, foster parents, childminders, and so on, within the most responsive local authorities. To have their own positions as lesbians recognized and secured within the workforce meant that some lesbians were able to feel more confident to challenge heterosexist practices within their workplaces. It also meant that they were supported in developing new ways of working with lesbian clients. Of course, the impact of the new policies was uneven, and it took some years for policy changes to produce significant changes in social work practice. However, securing an equal opportunities statement which includes sexual orientation marked a major advance in providing employment protection for lesbian and gay workers. Until lesbian workers felt that their jobs were secure, they were not in a position even to begin to examine the position of their clients (Davis 1983; Hillin 1985; Heathfield 1988).

Lesbian social workers have been concerned to develop a better social service response for lesbians, for both altruistic and pragmatic reasons. While lesbian clients are pathologized and discriminated against, so are lesbian social workers. Lesbian social workers aren't just social workers; they are also older lesbians, lesbian mothers, lesbians with disabilities, future lesbian foster-parents and lesbian co-parents, all of whom may have interactions with social services departments. Lesbian social workers have often been acutely aware of the inadequacies of the social work response to lesbian clients' needs, and because of this they have been motivated towards change.

At a series of national women and social work conferences in the late 1970s and early 1980s, lesbian social workers played an increasingly prominent role and began to set up local support groups. These groups gave more and more lesbian social workers the strength and confidence to raise issues of concern to lesbians within their agencies. (It should be remembered that, for the vast majority of local authorities, tackling discrimination against lesbians is not even on the agenda, and lesbian workers and clients in those authorities remain vulnerable.)

In the course of promoting positive initiatives towards lesbians, it became clear that to challenge heterosexism in social services departments and in social work practice meant challenging a substantial part of social work theory. It became apparent that it is not enough to move from oppression to acceptance; to establish non-discriminatory services for lesbians it is necessary to create a climate of equality for lesbians, which gives them the confidence to raise relevant issues within their workplaces. The scope for such developments depends on the political will of councillors and social services committees, as well as the broader pressures of national politics.

Since the mid-1980s, progressive developments in local government policy on lesbian and gay issues have come under sustained central government attack. The GLC was abolished in 1986, and local councils have been subjected to tighter financial and political constraints. In response to the propaganda attack on the 'loony left' image of radical Labour councils, particularly in London, the Labour Party leadership has become increasingly intolerant towards lesbian and gay issues. Under section 28 of the Local Government Act, 1988, local councils were forbidden to devote resources to the 'promotion' of homosexuality. The debate around the Human Fertilization Act in 1989 and 1990 encouraged popular prejudices against lesbians taking advantage of AID or IVF programmes (see Langan in this volume). All these developments have renewed the sense of insecurity of lesbian and gay workers and clients that was beginning to be allayed by the innovative equal opportunity policies of the early 1980s.

It is therefore of some importance that CCETSW has included anti-discriminatory practice competence within the criteria for qualification for the DipSW, as individual social workers and agencies may find themselves at variance with government policy and public opinion.

'Coming out' – implications for students, workers and clients

To 'come out' as a lesbian social worker, student or teacher, still carries risks. Judith Williams was a residential social worker who was sacked for being a lesbian in 1982, and her employer's policy of recruitment included this passage about prospective employees: 'Such persons should be mature, stable adults who identify with the conventional adult model normally accepted by society' (Davis 1983: 61). Social work education is presumably supposed to produce orthodox heterosexuals.

Even when working in more progressive agencies, lesbians may have great anxieties about being known as a lesbian. Some of these anxieties may be due to the way lesbians internalize or identify with homophobia, but most will arise from rational fears of colleagues', employers' and clients' responses. Local authorities' political complexions may change, and lesbians know that being 'out' in a progressive Labour-controlled local authority is different from being 'out' in a 'radical right' authority.

For black lesbian social workers there may be additional worries. The inter-relationship between racism and homophobia takes its toll on black lesbians, who have to struggle to find a way of personally negotiating both oppressions. The 'Gay Liberation Movement' and many white lesbians and gay men have placed great emphasis on the importance of 'coming out'. This is both because of the political significance of being visible, and for reasons of psychological wellbeing: 'Indeed, we see it as an essential part of building a positive and integrated self-concept, and reducing the tension between "me as others see me" and "me as I see myself" ' (Parry and Lightbown 1981: 164). This may be relevant for many white lesbians and gay men, but may not be applicable for some lesbian mothers or black lesbians, who may need to make clear choices in relation to where and with whom they are safe to be 'out'.

For example, great emphasis has been placed on being out with families. But black lesbians may not want to face possible rejection by their families, as they may feel them to be an important part of their culture and sense of themselves as black people. They may also experience their families as a 'safe place' in relation to racism. Not coming out, nevertheless, does place an additional strain on black lesbians, who are forced to hide aspects of their lives from those who are close to them (Carmen, Gail, Shaila and Pratibha 1984; GLC

1986a; Parmar 1989). Black lesbians cannot assume support from white lesbians and gay men, who are no more noted for their anti-racism than any other group.

At work, some black lesbians may well not want to be out, for fear of losing support from black colleagues. This is certainly the experience of many out white lesbians in relation to white colleagues. For some white lesbians in more secure positions, not being out can have other significance. In the words of a black social worker within my social services area office team: 'White lesbians can decide whether or not to be oppressed by being out or not; black women don't have that choice in relation to racism.' Although lesbian and gay social workers have won some concessions in securing their rights as employees, social work teachers and students are not so fortunate. The Association of University Teachers (AUT) and the National Association of Teachers in Further and Higher Education (NATFHE) both have incorporated sexual orientation into their equal opportunities policies, but have made little headway with the employers on these issues (NATFHE 1986; AUT 1987). Lesbian and gay social work teachers do not have a strong campaigning body within their unions, and they are in a far more vulnerable position than their NALGO counterparts. Institutions of higher education tend to lag behind local authorities in terms of implementing equal opportunities policies, even at the most basic level. As long as lesbian teachers feel insecure in their place of employment, they are unlikely to challenge heterosexism and homophobia on their courses, or to encourage their students to develop anti-discriminatory practices with lesbian clients.

Social work's traditional pathologizing of homosexuality still acts as a powerful influence on social work courses. The view that social workers should be mature, rational, emotionally and psychologically stable people, is in direct contrast to the stereotyped view of lesbians as immature (indeed arrested), irrational, emotionally and psychologically unstable. Social work education involves assessment of personal suitability for the job, as well as of academic and social work practice skills. As a result, students often feel constantly on their guard in relation to tutors, and many lesbian students, whether black or white, never come out on their social work courses.

On many social work courses, gender teaching is still at an embryonic stage (see Carter, Everitt and Hudson in this volume) and teaching about lesbians and gay men often non-existent. Much social work education is directly homophobic: 'Social work training courses do nothing to ensure the profession examines or is even made aware of its heterosexist assumptions' (Hillin 1985: 19). Developing the curriculum in this area means sifting through and reexamining much standard social work teaching, drawing on other material, developing our own material and using the experience and expertise of informed practitioners. The outstanding lesson that emerges from teaching in this area is that it is necessary that social work students and workers examine their own values, ideas, feelings and attitudes towards heterosexuality and homosexuality, before they are adequately equipped to work with men and women, heterosexual or homosexual. Social work students are no more and no less homophobic than anyone else. They may adopt a superficial understanding about working with lesbian clients, but unless they are able to explore their feelings about their own sexuality and that of others, they are likely to remain potentially dangerous, and the 'moral tyrants' referred to by Blyth and Hugman (1982: 65).

Positive developments in social work teaching about homosexuality will not happen until lesbian and gay teachers feel secure in their own institutions. The new DipSW requirements to develop non-discriminatory practice in teaching may help this process.

Practice implications

Older lesbians

Taking two areas of social work practice, work with older lesbians and lesbians and child protection work, we may begin to examine how we might use theory and skills to offer a 'good enough' social work intervention. Social workers have a responsibility to equip themselves to work with lesbians and gay men who come for, or are referred for, social work help, in such a way as facilitates the best possible outcome for the client.

Literature about human ageing and social work with older people tends to ignore issues of gender (see Hughes and Mtezuka in this volume). Writing that does incorporate a gender perspective into discussions about ageing ignores sexual orientation (Phillipson 1982; Willcocks 1983; Finch and Groves 1985). Writing that incorporates all four – social work, the ageing process, gender and sexual orientation – is scarce (Weeks 1981; Macdonald and Rich 1984; GLC and the GLC Gay Working Party 1985; Berger and Kelly 1986). Feminist writers have contributed greatly to the literature, looking at the inter-relationships between ageing, class, race, gender and sexual orientation (Macdonald and Rich 1984; Hemming 1985; Ford and Sinclair 1987).

Women form the greater part of the older population, and among that population a significant number will be lesbians. Older women are more vulnerable financially than men: 'For women . . . financial circumstances in old age are related not only to their previous employment history, but, crucially, also to their former marital status' (Finch and Groves 1985). Some older lesbians will have been or still be married, but many will have remained 'single', or lived with other women, whose earning capacities – in the main – will not have been equivalent to those of men. Social workers will therefore need to keep lesbian clients' economic circumstances in mind, as they may suffer disproportionate hardship.

Bereavement is not an unfamiliar predicament as people grow older, and some people may need skilled help to facilitate the grieving process (Worden 1983). Lesbians often experience additional pressures when they are bereaved. As their relationships are unrecognized by law, they are vulnerable in relation to joint property. They may never have openly acknowledged their relationship, and be ignored or even openly resented by families. They may feel there is nowhere sympathetic to go to talk through their loss. Given social work's reluctance to offer all older people proper counselling, older lesbians may be particularly vulnerable in respect to loss. Many older lesbians will not know about, or have access to, organizations such as the Gay Bereavement Project (Wertheimer 1987). Social services departments should offer counselling as a preventive mental health measure to older people who may be vulnerable in relation to bereavement; older lesbians may be a particularly vulnerable group.

Older lesbians have the experience of having lived through more oppressive times. They may have found ways of surviving in the world, without ever having 'come out'. There may be an enormous culture gap between a gender- and sexual-orientation-aware younger social worker and an older lesbian. We should not assume all lesbians want to 'come out', particularly to a social worker, but we need to work in ways that do not presume knowledge about the individual or make assumptions.

Older lesbians are often viewed as a pathetic, sad group. They may be more vulnerable in relation to economic status, bereavement and homophobia, but their different lifestyles may also be sources of strength. Some older lesbians may not have children to offer support, in the way that many heterosexuals have. However, many lesbians have networks of other adults, lesbian and heterosexual, that should be acknowledged by social workers.

For many heterosexual men and women, coping with the stigma of ageing is as hard as coping with the physical changes. But lesbians have always had to cope with stigmatization, in ways that might help them cope with the stigma of old age (Macdonald and Rich 1984).

Another possible area of strength is role flexibility (Berger and Kelly 1986). Lesbians are likely to have had more equal domestic relationships than heterosexual women, and may well be skilled in a wider range of domestic responsibilities, whether they have lived with others, with partners, or alone. If they are bereaved, they may be in a stronger position to continue with day-to-day existence, cooking, changing fuses, paying bills. This will vary from individual to individual, but in general lesbians will not have had such rigid division of domestic labour as their heterosexual counterparts.

When social workers are assessing the needs and appropriate services for an older lesbian, they need to be sensitive to the most appropriate resources. A client's sexual orientation is relevant information for a social worker to have, when looking at support systems or placements for an older person, but gaining and handling that information needs thought and sensitivity. An older lesbian, who can no longer manage at home with domicilliary input, may feel more comfortable living in a lesbian household, as an adult care placement, than with a heterosexual couple. Social services need to build up a wide range of options within their resources for older people, so they can offer the most appropriate placements to meet every individual's needs.

In some local authorities, home helps and other domicilliary care workers receive training in relation to sexual orientation. This has happened as a response to the need for training for staff working with people with Aids. All workers offering care to older people to facilitate them remaining at home, when this is their wish, need to confront their feelings about different sexualities and lifestyles. Otherwise they are not in a position to offer appropriate support and care to their clients.

Residential homes for older people will often have lesbian residents. Given the dominant heterosexual norm within most establishments, staff need to address the experience of the older lesbian and confront any homophobia that she may encounter. There are examples of this being done, to the benefit of the older lesbian (Davis 1983).

Given that social work is not renowned for its good work with older people in general, and older women specifically, older lesbians are likely to be particularly neglected, unless there is a real commitment to offer a good social work service to all older people irrespective of their sexual orientation. To do this will mean reassessing our theory, our policies, our resources and our social work practice.

Child protection

In the course of more than nine years in social services, as a practitioner and as a manager and supervisor, I came into contact with four lesbian families because the children were deemed 'at risk'. A number of points emerge from this limited number of cases that may help to illustrate how social work practice with lesbians and their children could be improved. The children had been abused in different ways, sexually, emotionally and physically. All of these families were different, some single lesbian mothers, some black lesbian mothers, some lesbian couples co-parenting children.

Working with these families exposed many myths surrounding lesbians as parents. First, there is a popular prejudice that lesbians are likely to abuse children sexually. Second, some believe that children of lesbian households will be unable to form a 'correct gender' identity or that they will develop 'gender confusion'. Third, others believe that lesbians are perverts and that a child in close proximity will inevitably be emotionally damaged. Another myth is that lesbians are not 'real women' and are therefore unable to mother. Others still think that children will be damaged by the stigma of living in a lesbian household.

However, psychiatric and psychological research in the United States and the United Kingdom contradicts these prejudiced assumptions on every count (Green 1978; Hoeffer 1981; Kirkpatrick *et al.* 1981; Golombok *et al.* 1983; Green *et al.* 1986). Research evidence shows that lesbians are equally as able to care for and bring up children as their heterosexual counterparts. However, just as some heterosexuals do not make good parents, some lesbians make inadequate parents and some – though very few – become potential abusers. For social workers to assess lesbian parents (where there has been a child care referral) they will have to be able to assess those individuals and their unique situation, and not rely on prejudiced assumptions.

The courts have often upheld popular prejudices about lesbian parenthood in their decisions to award custody to fathers on the grounds of the mother being lesbian in disputed cases (Rights of Women Lesbian Custody Group 1986; Radford and Cobley 1987). Evidence from the Lesbian Custody Project shows that social workers have been instrumental in lesbian mothers losing their children, through recommendations in their social inquiry reports (Radford and Cobley 1987). These social workers were guided by ignorance and prejudice, not by research evidence and knowledge. These actions have grave implications for mothers, but most significantly for the children, whose interests the social workers are meant to be safeguarding.

When we are working with lesbians who abuse their children, we need to have some general understanding of the pressures on women and the additional pressures on lesbians that may lead them to such behaviour (Brown 1986; Parton and Parton 1988). None of the women involved in our cases were worked with because they were lesbians, but all suffered from additional stresses from having to live with oppression and discrimination as the result of being lesbians. The women concerned, six in total, had legitimate anxieties about state intervention which were greater than those of most working-class and black women. They rightly assumed that their parenting capacities would be judged solely in relation to their sexual orientation. Thus, when social workers intervene in families in order to protect children, with the authority of the state, it is necessary to clarify why that intervention is taking place. This should be stated verbally and in written form, and thus openly shared with the clients. It should be explicitly recorded (with permission) that the sexual orientation of the carers is not the reason for intervention, and that it is not seen as a problem in itself. Social workers need to build a relationship of trust and openness with the parents to enable any positive work to take place in relation to these families and their children.

Even in this tiny sample of cases there was a variety of social workers involved, in terms of gender, race and sexual orientation. The quality of work done was dictated by the competence of the social work input, and the workers' ability to form appropriate, skilled relationships with the clients. The intervention outcomes were not affected by the sexual orientation of the workers, but by their abilities.

In working with these families it became apparent that there was a 'culture' gap (particularly in relation to class) between social workers and the clients. Whereas the social workers used phrases like 'co-parents' (for lesbians caring jointly for children), some clients felt the need to use terms like 'Mum' and 'Dad', so that they would be regarded as acceptable by the authorities. However, this indicated a desire to be accepted in a homophobic world, not 'gender confusion'. We should not assume a common language, or interpret others' use of words on face value.

Child protection work now involves mobilization of a wide variety of state agencies around any one case, including health, education, police and social services. However skilled and non-oppressive social work may be, social services departments can only influence, not control, other agencies. The experience of liaising with other agencies was varied, ranging from sensitive, clear, non-discriminatory input, through liberal stereotyping of the most unhelpful nature, to outright homophobia. When referring lesbian carers to specialist agencies in relation to child abuse, social services departments should assess the attitudes of those agencies towards lesbians. Unless this is done, they are not safeguarding the interests of children, as they will be unlikely to work effectively with the families.

In the field of child protection it is common for workers to be afraid that parents may damage them after children have been removed. Lesbian social workers' fears are often focused on the client misusing information about their sexual orientation and this may become a factor in whether she chooses to be 'out' at work.

The dangers of negative and positive stereotyping have been excellently demonstrated in the Tyra Henry inquiry (London Borough of Lambeth 1987). The inquiry describes how the black Afro-Caribbean grandmother was seen as a type, a positive stereotype of an all-coping indestructible matriarch, not as an individual. Positive stereotyping happened in one of our cases, where the commitment to lesbian parenting, for a short time, predominated over the interests of the child. This mother's activities were seen in a prejudiced and distorted way: 'I thought that was normal for lesbians.' Any stereotyping, where people see a particular individual as a type, will not be in anyone's interest, particularly children's.

To offer 'good enough' support to a family that may be under stress, the social services department needs to have resources that welcome and validate lesbians' families. This is a necessary backdrop to facilitate social workers' intervention.

Concluding thoughts

Both social workers and clients live in a world that hates, fears, and is fascinated by, homosexuality. Social work with lesbians takes place in this context. Lesbians are not clients because they are lesbians, but because they may need social work intervention for a wide variety of reasons, just like heterosexuals. The very fact that social work enters the 1990s in a state of crisis creates the possibility of reviewing its practices in relation to lesbians. To ensure a satisfactory standard it is necessary to review, deconstruct and reconstruct our theory, policies and practice in the light of class, race, gender, disability and sexual orientation. We need to develop competent social work on the basis of non-prejudicial knowledge and non-oppressive practice. This is a long road. To do this, social work educators, social workers and students need the support of CCETSW, their management and institutions. This support will only be gained through hard-fought battles. But at the end of the day we must secure all clients the right to non-oppressive, non-discriminatory social work practice.

Acknowledgements

I wish to acknowledge the support and help given to me in producing this chapter by Mary Langan and Maggie Wilkinson. I also want to acknowledge what I have learnt from lesbian colleagues, students and clients over the last twelve years.

References

Association of University Teachers (1987), *Ensuring equal opportunities for university staff and students from ethnic minorities* (London: AUT).

Berger, R. M. and Kelly, J. J. (1986), 'Working with homosexuals of the older population', *Social Casework* 67, 4, pp. 203–10.

Blyth, M. J. and Hugman, B. (1982), 'Social work education and probation', in R. Bailey and P. Lee (eds), *Theory and Practice in Social Work* (Oxford: Blackwell) pp. 61–77.

Boston Lesbian Psychologies Collective (1987), *Lesbian Psychologies* (Chicago: University of Illinois Press).

Brook, E. and Davis, A. (1985), *Women, the Family and Social Work* (London: Tavistock).

Brown, C. (1986), 'Child abuse – a failure of social work practice?' *Spare Rib* 161, p. 12.

Carmen, Gail, Shaila and Pratibha (1984), 'Becoming visible', *Feminist Review* 17, pp. 53–72.

CCETSW (1989), 'DipSW requirements and regulations for the Diploma in Social Work', paper 30 (London: CCETSW).

Christopher, E. (1980), *Sexuality and Birth Control in Social and Community Work* (London: Maurice Temple Smith).

Dale, J. and Foster, P. (1986), *Feminists and State Welfare* (London: Routledge and Kegan Paul).

Davis, L. (1983), *Sex and the Social Worker* (London: Heinemann).

Dominelli, L. and McLeod, E. (1989), *Feminist Social Work* (London: Macmillan).

Fanon, F. (1967), *Black Skins, White Masks* (New York: Grove Press).

Faraday, A. (1981), 'Liberating lesbian research', in K. Plummer (ed.), *The Making of the Modern Homosexual* (London: Hutchinson) pp. 112–29.

Finch, J. and Groves, D. (1985), 'Old girl, old boy: gender divisions in social work with the elderly', in E. Brook and A. Davis (eds), *Women, the Family and Social Work* (London: Tavistock) pp. 92–111.

Ford, J. and Sinclair, P. (1987), *Sixty Years On: Women Talk about Old Age* (London: The Women's Press).

Gagnon, J. H. and Simon, W. (1973), *Sexual Conduct* (Chicago: Aldine).

GLC (1986a), *Tackling Heterosexism* (London: GLC Women's Committee).

GLC (1986b), *Danger: Heterosexism at Work* (London: Spider Publications).
GLC and the GLC Gay Working Party (1985), *Changing the World, London Charter for Gay and Lesbian Rights* (London: Strategic Policy Unit).
Golombok, S., Spencer, A. and Rutter, M. (1983), 'Children in lesbian and single parent households: psychosexual and psychiatric appraisal', *Journal of Child Psychology and Psychiatry* 24, 4.
Green, R. (1978), 'Sexual identity of thirty-seven children raised by homosexual or transvestite parents', *American Journal of Psychiatry* June, pp. 135–6.
Green, R. *et al.* (1986), 'Lesbian mothers and their children: a comparison with solo parent heterosexual mothers and their children', *Archives of Sexual Behaviour* 15 (12), pp. 167–84.

Hanmer, J. and Statham, D. (1988), *Women and Social Work* (London: Macmillan).
Hart, T. and Richardson, D. (eds) (1981), *The Theory and Practice of Homosexuality* (London: Routledge and Kegan Paul).
Heathfield, M. (1988), 'The youth work response to lesbian and gay youth', *Youth and Policy* 23, pp. 19–22.
Hemming, S. (1985), *A Wealth of Experience* (London: Pandora Press).
Hillin, A. (1985), 'When you stop hiding your sexuality', *Social Work Today* 4, pp. 18–19.
Hoeffer, B. (1981), 'Children's acquisition of sex role behaviour in lesbian-mother families', *American Journal of Orthopsychiatry* 51, 3.
Howe, D. (1986), 'The segregation of women and their work in the personal social services', *Critical Social Policy* 15, 5, 3, pp. 21–35.

Kirkpatrick, M., Smith, M. and Roy, R. (1981), 'Lesbian mothers and their children: a comparative survey', *American Journal of Orthopsychiatry* 5, 13, pp. 545–51.
Kitzinger, C. (1987), *The Social Construction of Lesbianism* (London: Saga Publications).

Labour Campaign for Lesbian and Gay Rights (1986), *Legislation for Lesbian and Gay Rights: A Manifesto*, August (London: Labour Campaign for Lesbian and Gay Rights).
London Borough of Lambeth (1987), *Whose Child? The Report of the Panel Appointed to Inquire Into the Death of Tyra Henry* (London Borough of Lambeth).

Macdonald, B. and Rich, C. (1984), *Look Me in the Eye* (London: The Women's Press).
McKay, J. (1984), 'History of Nalgo's policies on lesbian and gay rights', NALGO National Equal Opportunities Committee Seminar, January (unpublished).

NATFHE (1986) *Sexual Orientation. An Equal Opportunities Discussion Paper* (London: NATFHE).

Parmar, P. (1989), 'Black lesbians' in A. Phillips and J. Rakusen (eds), *The New Our Bodies Ourselves* (Penguin), pp. 221–2.
Parry, G. and Lightbown, R. (1981), in Hart and Richardson 1981, pp. 159–64.
Parton, C. (1990), 'Women, gender oppression and child abuse', in The Violence Against Children Study Group, *Taking Child Abuse Seriously* (London: Unwin Hyman), pp. 41–62.
Parton, C. and Parton, N. (1988), 'Women, the family and child protection', *Critical Social Policy* 24, 8, pp. 38–49.
Pearson, G., Threseder, J. and Yelloly, M. (1988), *Social Work and the Legacy of Freud* (London: Macmillan).
Phillipson, C. (1982), *Capitalism and the Construction of Old Age* (London: Macmillan).
Plummer, K. (1975), *Sexual Stigma, an Interactionist Account* (London: Routledge and Kegan Paul).

Radford, J. and Cobley, J. (1987), 'Lesbian custody project on social work reports', *Rights of Women Bulletin*, May.
Richardson, D. (1981), 'Lesbian identities', in Hart and Richardson 1981, pp. 111–24.
Rights of Women Lesbian Custody Group (1986), *Lesbian Mothers' Legal Handbook* (London: The Women's Press).
Ryan, J. (1983), 'Psychoanalysis and women loving women', in S. Cartledge and J. Ryan (eds), *Sex and Love, New Thoughts on Old Contradictions* (London: The Women's Press), pp. 196–209.

Tobin, A. (1990), 'Lesbianism and the Labour Party: the GLC experience', *Feminist Review* 34, pp. 56–66.
Trevithick, P. and Ryan, J. (1988), 'Lesbian workshop' in S. Krzowski and P. Land (eds), *In Our Experience* (London: The Women's Press) pp. 102–13.

Weeks, J. (1981), 'The problems of older homosexuals' in Hart and Richardson 1981, pp. 177–84.
Wertheimer, A. (1987), 'Mourning in secret', *New Society* 80, 1268, pp. 8–9.
Willcocks, D. (1983), 'Gender and the care of elderly people in Part III accommodation', paper presented at the British Society of Gerontology annual conference at the University of Liverpool.
Wilson, E. (1977), *Women and the Welfare State* (London: Tavistock).
Wolff, C. (1971), *Love Between Women* (London: Duckworth).
Worden, J. W. (1983), *Grief Counselling and Grief Therapy* (London: Tavistock).

Yelloly, M. A. (1980), *Social Work Theory and Psychoanalysis* (London: Van Nostrand Reinhold).

12 *Social work and older women: where have older women gone?*

Beverley Hughes and Melody Mtezuka

Introduction: the rise of critical gerontology

If coverage in academic literature is a valid measure of importance, then older women must be singularly unimportant. Until recently, the subject of older women was conspicuous only by its absence from sociological, gerontological, feminist and social work literature. Early investigations of the community and institutional life of older people exposed poverty and disadvantage in the daily lives of many old people (Townsend 1957; Tunstall 1966). Yet despite this evidence of the need for further empirical and theoretical research into the social lives and structural position of old people, it was left to one or two tenacious sociologists to continue this exploration (Phillipson 1972; Townsend 1981; Walker 1981). Most official literature was permeated with images of old age as a time of decline and dependency. It was generally assumed that dependency, whether physical, mental, social or economic, was a natural and inevitable consequence of the biological process of ageing. This construction of old age was legitimated by the theory of disengagement which saw the withdrawal of older people from social roles and the mainstream of social life not only as desirable for older people themselves but also functional for society (Cumming and Henry 1961). This ideology permeated social policy towards older people on both sides of the Atlantic for many years.

Towards the end of the 1970s, a coherent theoretical challenge to disengagement theory began to emerge, and since then critical gerontology has developed considerably its analysis of ageism under capitalism (Phillipson and Walker 1986). Ageism is the social process through which negative images of and attitudes towards older people, based solely on the characteristics of old age itself, result in discrimination. This can be observed in the relative disadvantage experienced by older people as a group in a number of social, economic and other dimensions of life. Critical gerontology rejects the notion that the experiences of old people derive essentially from the biological process of ageing. It looks instead to the social construction of ageing as the primary reason for the marginalization of old people. It has focused until recently on charting and explaining the basic economic, social, health and other disadvantages experienced by older people as a group. However, the study of differentiation *among* old people is a recent phenomenon. It is significant that the revelation (as it must surely be termed), that: 'the world of the very old is . . . a woman's world' (Peace 1986: 61) was made first, not by feminist writers, but by critical gerontologists.

The failure of feminism

Despite the fact that older women constitute a substantial minority of the total population and a majority of the population older than 65, feminists have paid them little attention. Macdonald and Rich have observed that 'so far the women's movement has resonated with its silence on the subject of the status of old women' (Macdonald and Rich 1984: 53). Feminism may be fairly accused not only of neglecting older women, but of reinforcing both the ageism and the sexism which affect their lives. Three characteristics of the women's movement have contributed to its failure in relation to older women. First, one of the central features of the women's movement has been its campaign to construct images of womanhood which emphasize the strength and power of women. Women have been encouraged to shed the victim role in domestic, economic, social, and political life, to be assertive and to reject the images of weakness and dependency. But what meaning do these images offer older women? By failing to embrace a multiplicity of images of womanhood, which would include and validate the frailty and dependency of some older women, feminists have cut themselves off from their own futures. Older women are given no place in 'the strong chain' that links new women together. Rich has argued that 'The evidence is all around that youth is bonded within patriarchy in the enslavement of older women' (Macdonald and Rich 1984: 39). Indeed, she goes on to assert that the ageism which has until very recently characterized the women's movement 'must be some indication of the degree to which we have all internalised male values' (Macdonald and Rich 1984: 36).

A second feature of feminism is the assumption that the issues facing older women are the same as those facing young women, and the conviction that the problems of older women will inevitably be solved by the changes achieved by and for young women. This view takes no account either of the structured dependency experienced by old people or of the consequences for women of growing old in a society in which youth is highly valued. The women's movement has failed to acknowledge divergence and differentiation amongst women and, through its treatment of older women, has reinforced the values of an ageist society. Most books on the condition of women in society have not included any acknowledgement of the specific oppression of older women. For example Stacey boldly asserts the women's movement's relevance to all women:

> Those of us who have understood feminism in collectivist rather than individualistic terms have a concept of womanhood which embraces all women in all conditions in all places' (Stacey 1983: 10).

The book in which this is written contains chapters on a variety of conditions of womanhood, none of which embrace old age (Gamarnikow *et al.* 1983).

Third, in so far as feminist writers have acknowledged older women, it has been as objects needing the care of younger women (for example, Finch 1984). It is true that the responsibility of caring for older women tends to fall on younger women, either in the home or in institutions. However, focus on these issues has not been balanced by an interest in older women themselves, either in terms of their experiences as recipients of care, or in relation to the strategies older women adopt to meet the challenges of ageism and sexism. Evers (1983) and more recently Ford and Sinclair (1989) have begun to redress this imbalance, and to challenge the portrayal of older women as important for the feminist movement only in so far as they constitute work objects for younger women.

Social work literature: a sad case of neglect

Social work texts, especially those attempting to develop alternative or radical practice, have not generally applied their new thinking to work with old people. Furthermore, many of the social work texts examining gender issues have also failed to include older women in their analyses of women as clients, carers, and practitioners (for example, Hanmer and Statham 1988).

In so far as elderly people do appear, the images portrayed tend to be consistent with ageist stereotypes. In addition, in so far as they fail to acknowledge differentiation amongst old people, these images also embody sexist, racist and classist assumptions. Most importantly, social work literature does not reflect the fact that the majority of old people are women. Finch and Groves have criticized the images of older women in social work literature on the grounds that:

> [They] rarely take account of the fact that the majority of the very old elderly are female, 'infantilize' elderly people, show examples of traditional gender behaviour as fostered by social workers, uphold living arrangements based on traditional family forms and portray the stereotyped 'lonely widow' (Finch and Groves 1985: 109).

While there are signs of innovation by some practitioners working with older people, the general attitude of academic social work to older people has been one of neglect (for an example of the more positive trends see Walker 1985).

Ideologies and social constructions

Older women experience ageism and sexism. Thus, they occupy contradictory positions, being united with and divided from old men, and united with and divided from other women. Perhaps the contradictory nature of their position accounts in part for the fact that older women have not been owned or acknowledged as important constituents of either the elderly or the female populations. Yet, the connections between ageism and sexism are profound and mutually reinforcing. Indeed, MacDonald and Rich argue that 'To begin to understand ageism is to recognise that it is a point of convergence for many other repressive forces' (MacDonald and Rich 1984: 61).

Ageism and sexism are connected in two ways. First, the impact of ageing on women has implications for the extent to which old women can conform to the image of womanhood propagated by sexism. A woman not only loses the physical attractiveness ascribed to the ideal woman, but also the prescribed social roles of caring for the family. Indeed, she may need care herself and, as the carer becomes the cared-for, a role reversal underlines the failure of the older woman to conform to the stereotype of womanhood. Thus, passage into old age increases the potential for dissonance with social norms of womanhood and femininity.

Second, an old woman evokes primeval images of women as mystics and witches, derived from woman's proximity to (and men's alienation from) the processes of nature. MacDonald and Rich construct a concept of ageism as 'a powerful force itself, one deeply rooted in Western man's unconscious fears' (MacDonald and Rich 1984: 61). Women's control over natural forces is associated, through childbirth, with all life-processes, including death. Thus, ageism can also be seen as the manifestation of the most atavistic prejudices against women.

While ageism and sexism run common threads through the lives of older women as a group, the extent to which other factors either aggravate or ameliorate these effects is an important source of differentiation among older women. Thus, being working class or black imposes a greater complexity and potential for contradiction in the lives of older women and, at the same time, may result in life experiences and perceptions which are qualitatively different from older women who are middle class or white. Finally, it is arguable that social class and life history are the sources of the most dramatic differentiation amongst older women. Yet there is no satisfactory means of ascribing social class to older women. Occupational classification, of dubious value for younger women, is even less valid in assigning social class to older women.

Older women as a social group: factors which unite older women

Socio-economic characteristics

> Elderly people dominate the poverty statistics and have done ever since the systematic studies of Charles Booth. . . . But poverty is not evenly distributed among the elderly and gender is one of the clearest lines along which the economic and social experience of old age is divided (Walker 1987: 178).

As a group, old women are more likely than men to be very old, very poor, single or widowed and living alone. Women's greater longevity, with a life expectancy at 60 of 21 years, compared to 16 years for men, accounts only in part for these differences. As a much greater proportion of women than men survive to advanced old age, so the likelihood of widowhood and of living alone increases. In addition, the present generation of old women contains a significant proportion of single women, the legacy of two world wars which killed or disabled many men.

However, the poverty and financial instability of old women are less the results of biology and war, and more the consequences of oppression. Older women experience a more extreme version of the social and economic discrimination common to women of every age, and the difficulties of older women are compounded by retirement policies and pension schemes (Groves 1987; Walker 1987).

The social circumstances of older women are markedly different from those of older men. Older women are more likely to be single or widowed, and this tendency increases significantly with age. At age 75 years and over, for example, 80 per cent of women, but only

39 per cent of men are unmarried (that is, never married, widowed or divorced) (OPCS 1983). Older women are also more likely to be living alone – 58 per cent at age 75+, compared to 26 per cent of men in this age group (Family Policy Studies Centre 1988).

Finally, while older women living alone appear – in terms of household income and living situation – to be the most disadvantaged sub-group within the retired population, Walker has warned that official statistics may 'underestimate the poverty of elderly married women' (Walker 1987: 182). This occurs partly because it is assumed that the household income of a couple is distributed equally between male and female partners, and partly because the method of compilation of figures fails to identify women's more limited access to pensions in their own right or via their husbands.

Health

The differences in health between men and women at all ages are complex (Markides 1989). On the one hand, up to the age of 65, men in each social class are twice as likely as women to die (Townsend and Davidson 1988). On the other hand, women in old age appear to experience more health problems than men. Older women living in the community, especially those living alone, are more likely to report long-standing chronic conditions and, as a consequence, experience greater loss of mobility and other physical limitations (Hunt 1978; OPCS 1982). Men living in the community appear to be more likely to fall into one of two categories: either very well and fit, or acutely ill. Women constitute the majority of institutional populations, and are much less well and able than male residents/patients.

It might be expected that the impact of different patterns of mortality, longevity and illness among men and women in old age would be reflected in different levels and patterns of dependency and capacity for self-care. However, the evidence suggests that the extent to which men and women report their capacities to undertake activities of daily living is influenced not only by physical limitation due to illness, but also by gender-derived expectations about what men and women can or ought to be able to do for themselves. Thus, while ability was shown to be age-related, several studies have reported that, despite greater mobility and less chronic illness among men, they are twice as likely to report the inability to wash clothes, prepare meals, or do small sewing jobs (Hunt 1978).

Finally, the attitudes and expectations of old women and old men in relation to health and ill-health appear to be different. These differences may be reflected both in the extent of reported ill-health and in expressed satisfaction. Several studies have noted how older women have a greater tendency, in spite of experiencing long-standing illness, to report general satisfaction with their health. Thus, women live at home, often alone, with problems and 'disabilities that might cause men to go into institutions' (Hunt 1978: 69). Evers (1985) suggests that older women may be expected to be able to cope with the consequences of disability better than men. However, it is also likely that, after a lifetime of socially-constructed dependency of all forms, older women themselves have low expectations and more easily accept the consequences of disability. Conversely, they may have also learned that they have to simply get on and make the best of things, which they do, but often at no small cost to themselves.

Social experience of womanhood

Women progress towards old age with a wealth of accumulated experience of what it is like to be a woman in this society. In terms of the experience of relationships with men, and of roles of dependant, wife, mother and daughter, the lives of different women may be touched by common themes and common experiences which are brought into old age.

Hemmings identifies the struggles of marriage, and the experience of subjugation perceived by married women, as a common theme amongst the diverse contributors to her book:

> What, then, despite all our differences in background, are our shared experiences? Marriage! It comes up over and over again. . . . Some of the contributors chronicle a sharing of love, care, responsibilities: most tell of agonizing incompatibilities, or a give and take which turned out mainly at the women's expense. Even in reasonably 'good' marriages, women describe how they have for years suppressed their own needs and intellect in order to preserve their husband's sense of self (Hemmings 1985: 7).

Whether married or not, women are ascribed the role of carer throughout life and, through this role, put their own needs, wishes and aspirations behind those of their partners, children and families. Yet, paradoxically, women's enforced dependency and carer role have resulted in many women having control and responsibility within the private domain of home life. Women's lives within this sphere have been characterized by the need to balance the demands of children, partner and parents; by having to calm the troubled waters of turbulent emotional family life; by the pressure of coping not only emotionally, but also economically; by having to be seen to 'manage' at whatever level of social hierarchy a woman lives. The image women have of themselves as they enter old age is heavily influenced by the social construction of womanhood and the roles and duties it embodies.

Factors which differentiate older women

Race and culture

Although there is an emerging body of expertise, minority ethnic communities are still marginalized in social work policy and practice (Glendenning 1979; Norman 1985). In 1988, when the Wagner report – a major review of residential services for elderly people – was published, the chair of the committee commented that she was:

> most disappointed by our failure to deal satisfactorily with the needs of the ethnic minority communities whom we recognise to be particularly ill-served by the residential sector (Gaffaney 1988: 2).

The failure of the residential sector to meet the needs of black older people is replicated in all aspects of social work practice and service delivery.

Most social work literature on elderly people is written as though Britain was a purely white society (Rowlings 1981; Marshall 1983). Even critical analysts such as Walker (1987) and Finch and Groves (1983), who have begun to distinguish the specific effects of ageism and sexism, have failed to consider racism. It is possible that white British writers feel unqualified to make observations about minority groups. While this defensive position may be valid, it nevertheless conceals the racism inherent in British society.

The covert racism experienced by minority ethnic groups can also be seen in the way black and minority ethnic communities are often perceived as a homogeneous group. This perception negates the different historical, social and cultural experiences of the diverse cultural groups, as well as the different economic and social reasons for migration to Britain, with varying consequences for the now-older people. For example, Fenton (1988) points out that whereas many immigrants from the New Commonwealth and Pakistan (NCWP) were single men who remained isolated from their families for many years, there was a higher proportion of female immigrants from the Caribbean and West Africa.

Many older Afro-Caribbean women came to Britain to join husbands, but many more came as single people. They found jobs which white workers were no longer willing to do, such as night- and day-time cleaning, canteen work, laundry work, 'an extension of the work we had done under colonisation in the Caribbean' (Bryan *et al.* 1985: 25).

For many, coming to Britain was intended to provide a better future for their children and/or themselves (Hemmings 1985). There was a push towards high employment activity among the Afro-Caribbean women (Glendenning and Pearson 1988). However, the jobs secured were generally unlikely to provide financial independence, with consequent lack of financial and material security in old age (Norman 1985; Fenton 1988; Glendenning and Pearson 1988).

The circumstances of many of these women meant that even when they suffered from chronic ill-health, for example through diabetes or high blood pressure, they had to carry on working (Fenton 1988; Townsend and Davidson 1988). Furthermore, illnesses with a genetic component, such as sickle cell anaemia, added to chronic ill-health and debility, particularly as the National Health Service has failed to provide adequate screening programems.

> the Health Service is central to our lives, we cannot avoid using it. . . . Because we are working-class women, we have no access to the growing number of private or natural alternatives, so favoured by those with the financial resources to go elsewhere. But above all, because we are *Black* women, whether we seek treatment within or outside the NHS, we invariably find ourselves dealing with a profession which is fundamentally patriarchal and racist (Bryan *et al.* 1985: 90).

Afro-Caribbean women, therefore, are likely to have experienced a harsh and precarious existence with little opportunity to provide for security in old age.

Women from the Indian sub-continent are especially vulnerable to being stereotyped through the use of the collective term 'Asian'. While this term may be useful in order to distinguish this minority group from others, it can also obscure the complex linguistic, religious and cultural patterns of each sub-group. Not all Asians originate from the Indian sub-continent. There is a sizeable number of settlers from Uganda and Kenya who have been exposed to varied socialization patterns. Nevertheless, all Asians as a group experience 'a host community not always very sympathetic to their cultural traditions' (Mooneram 1979: 51).

While there is evidence that a high proportion of younger Asian women as a group are now in paid employment, it is more likely that older women from particular minority ethnic groups have been involved exclusively in domestic duties or homework throughout their lives. Older women of Pakistani or Bangladeshi origin, for example, may have been less active in outside paid employment, and may therefore be more isolated, than their Afro-Caribbean or African-Asian counterparts. The myth of the extended family support system assumes that Asian people in this country are able to care for their old relatives as well as for their children within the same household (Glendenning 1979). However, British housing stock and immigration policies have led to the breakdown of extended family support systems. Overcrowding makes it more difficult for adult children to execute family responsibilities toward ageing parents. Statistics show that households with a head from the NCWP are seven times more likely to be overcrowded and fourteen times more likely to be extremely overcrowded than those households whose head was born in Britain (Whitehead 1988). Thus older people find themselves in a hostile society and an alien culture. Tensions can arise when an elderly parent expects to be able to live with and be cared for by an adult son or daughter, whose family may be unable or unwilling to provide such care.

Older people may experience a loss of status in the cultural traditions of family life and can ultimately be perceived, and perceive themselves, as a burden (Norman 1985). For older people from NCWP, there is additional financial pressure, as family members now have to sign a declaration that they will not call upon state funding for their elders. Many black older women experience isolation and despair, loss of position and status, compounded by poverty, bad housing and low income.

However, an understanding of the impact of individual, institutional and cultural racism on the lives of black older women has to be integrated with a commitment to avoiding stereotypes (Dominelli 1989). While the experience of ageism, sexism and poverty for black older women will be different from that of their white sisters, these dimensions of their lives must be understood not only for black older women as a group but also for each individual. Black older women too can step outside the boundaries of cultural norms and expectations in their struggle for liberation (Ford and Sinclair 1987).

Social class

It is clear that those characteristics of life which derive from social class – income and wealth, education, housing, employment, lifestyle and values – exert a powerful determining influence on quality of life in old age. Indeed, social class:

> Defines the resources available, it determines attitudes and habits and it has shaped the personal biography of which old age is but the continuing development (Ford and Taylor 1981: 332).

The concept of the 'feminization of poverty' reflects the fact that women as a group have been, and are increasingly, at greater risk of poverty than men (Glendinning and Millar 1987). Within the elderly population, the socio-economic characteristics of old women and old men are in even more stark contrast. However, it is also clear that the conditions of life experienced by older women are strongly mediated, for better or worse, by the class-determined characteristics of their lives as younger women.

Working-class women are more likely to have experienced low income or poverty throughout life (Walker 1987); to have limited access to pension provision (Groves 1987); to have lived, and continue in old age to live, in poor housing conditions (Townsend 1979); and to have been disadvantaged by the discriminatory assumptions which underpin state income maintenance systems (Callender 1987). Conversely, women from the professional, middle and upper classes are more likely to have access to resources acquired throughout life, with which to offset the consequences of enforced retirement and female economic dependency.

The association between social class and health has been firmly established. Disability has also been shown to be class-related. In a brief review of literature, Wilkin and Hughes conclude:

> There is evidence that health status in old age is more a product of experiences throughout life, than of old age *per se*, and that people from social classes I and II are less likely than those from poorer backgrounds to suffer the most debilitating conditions (Wilkin and Hughes 1987: 164).

Indeed, the chance of reaching old age is closely related to social class. In her review of a number of studies examining the mortality rates and health status of different social groups, Whitehead reports that 'the risk of death for lower occupational groups in the 1980's was much higher than that of the highest occupational classes at every stage of life' (Whitehead 1988: 236). While the particular patterns of class–mortality relationship were different for men and women, the general trend within both sex groups was the same. The experience and perception of health is not only worse for women in lower socio-economic groups but there is evidence that the gap between the lowest and highest socio-economic groups in terms of health status is widening (Whitehead 1988). Furthermore, the health care system appears to have little effect on overcoming class differentials in health, even in relation to treatable illnesses associated with poverty.

Apart from socio-economic and health factors, there are likely to be other differences between older women in the lower and higher social class groups, although research and evidence is sparse. Older women in lower social classes are more likely to be widowed, and widowed earlier, although they may fare better in terms of close proximity of adult offspring as a potential source of support. Expectations of older women – in terms of quality of life according to a number of indices including health, security, income and access to services – tend to be lower for women whose whole-life experiences have been characterized by poverty and inequality. This is a particularly important factor for service providers and practitioners working with older women.

Life history

So far we have been concerned to identify the structural social factors which either collectivize or differentiate older women. Older women, perhaps inevitably, have been portrayed predominantly as victims of various forms of social and economic oppression. In charting the sources of oppression we may inadvertently validate those images of older women we are seeking to challenge. The concepts of life history and personal biography enable us to redress the balance.

The testimony of older women proclaims that if they are victims, they are not passive victims, and if they are oppressed it is not for want of struggle (Matthews 1979; Macdonald and Rich 1984; Hemmings 1985; Ford and Sinclair 1987). The process by which people internalize social constructions is complex and the impact of ideology on different individuals is diverse (Leonard 1984). Some older women internalize the social norms associated with womanhood in old age, while others reject them. Evers (1985) has suggested that personal adaptation to old age, and to the concept of dependency in particular, depends less on health, class and family relationships and more on self-image, especially perceived purposefulness and control over life, derived from individual life history. Her interim paper identified two groups of older women – passive responders and active initiators. Women categorized as passive responders were those who already defined themselves as dependent and in need of care, irrespective of physical health. The earlier lives of these older women were characterized by unpaid care work, usually exclusively for the family. Active initiators, on the other hand, subjectively defined themselves as independent and in control of their daily lives. These women had generally worked outside the home, had more hobbies and interests, or engaged in political activity when they were younger.

We would do well to remember that the women in this generation of old people are survivors and that their lives, and their survival, have inevitably involved the surmounting of personal and social challenges throughout this century. As their personal biographies reveal, older women are endowed with resources and experiences which are not sufficiently acknowledged. Hemmings advocates the investigation of personal testimony as means of 'conscious revelation of shared experiences which enables us to rise above the level of "victim" so often ascribed to middle-aged and older women' (Hemmings 1985: 2). Thus, personal biographies do not negate the common experiences of oppression by individualizing them, but rather they articulate the ways in which many women, in their earlier lives, confronted the consequences of oppression, and often did so collectively with other women (Hemmings 1985). An understanding of personal biography and life history is essential to understanding how different older women interpret, negotiate and respond to old age.

Current policy and practice

Community care or community warehousing?

There have been many excellent reviews of the implications of the current policy of community care for women as low paid or unpaid carers of infirm older people (Finch and Groves 1980; Wright 1986). Here, however, we examine the implications of this policy for the older woman herself. As we have observed, older women are more likely than men to suffer some degree of incapacity, especially if they are very old, poor or black. Thus, the policy of community care, whatever that means in practice, is more likely to impinge on the lives of older women.

Community care was defined by Griffiths (1988) as the identification and generation of community resources and their integration with the services of family, neighbours, voluntary agencies and the private sector to create packages of care to meet the needs of individual old people. The Griffiths report on community care, adopted by the government in 1989, has two important consequences for older people (HMSO 1989). Firstly, there is concern that the level of support envisaged by the government falls far below what professionals and consumers themselves would regard as necessary to maintain a frail older person at home with an acceptable level of risk and a good quality of life. For example, the Audit Commission, in a costing exercise designed to demonstrate that community care is cheaper than residential care for severely disabled old people, based its calculation on a package of 'intensive community care' support services which consisted of 9 home help hours, 5 meals on wheels and 2 day care attendances per week (Audit Commission 1985: 15).

This level of care cost £45 per week at 1982/83 prices, compared to £60 for residential care. The package, however, consists only of a low level of basic services, and includes no provision for respite care, night-sitting services, laundry facilities or social worker time.

If an old woman had to rely on this level of support she would be impoverished in terms of stimulation, social contact, and recreation; she would be forced to live at a standard of material and environmental comfort which would deteriorate rapidly over time. She would not be *cared* for in the community, but rather warehoused in the community.

The second important consequence of community care is the potential impact on the relationships between older women and their spouses, offspring, relatives and friends in general, and their adult daughters, in particular. In the context of a minimalist approach to the provision of state sector services, the trend is towards ever more care being provided by family members, and mostly by women. After a lifetime of caring for others, many older women are acutely conscious of the danger of becoming a burden for another woman (Ford and Sinclair 1987; 1989). Many express a wish to remain close to, but independent of, their children. Older women who need care and who cannot claim support services in their own right may be forced into a carer/cared-for relationship which brings additional complexities to their position as older women. The potential for conflict between older women and adult daughters who are locked in such a relationship, with its role reversal and symbolic power differential, is considerable (Brody *et al.* 1984).

Social work practice

Social work has not only failed to challenge ageism and its implicit assumptions of assumed homogeneity, it appears to have embraced these values. Furthermore, social work and social service provision have failed to identify the particular needs of the *majority* of old people – that is, older women – and, within that group, have not recognized the diversity related to social class, race and life history.

Within many social services departments (and hospitals and health authorities) work with old people appears to be regarded as less important, less skilled, less stressful and less complex than work with other groups such as children and mentally ill people (Bowl 1986). Assessment is usually limited to assessment of the need and criteria for provision of practical aids (Means 1981). Intervention which follows assessment is usually short term and characterized by surveillance rather than direct work with old people and their families to achieve change. A wider perspective on relationships and family dynamics in the lives of old people appears to be absent from the professional view of social work with old people, which effectively excludes longer term work, casework and groupwork (Finch and Groves 1985).

While policy relating to service development has tended to assume that all older people are the same, there is evidence that in their day-to-day work, social workers and other service providers apply implicit gender assumptions as to the kinds of services that older men and older women, respectively, need.

> While social workers, along with most other people may be gender-blind in their explicit thinking about the elderly, they still can (and, it appears, often do) operate with implicit gender assumptions in their dealings with elderly clients (Finch and Groves 1985: 97).

In terms of the provision of specific services, there appear to be gender-related patterns emerging from social workers' role as gate-keepers of resources. In the context of low levels of service provision – only 9 per cent of the total elderly population receive regular home help service – there is growing evidence that men have greater access to some services despite their generally better health and mobility (Hunt 1978; OPCS 1982). A similar trend emerges in relation to male and female carers (Charlesworth *et al.* 1984). Peace conjectures that the basis for observed gender-based patterns of service provision lies in the belief that 'the hidden rules concerning role divisions based on gender do exist, even in extreme old age' (Peace 1986: 71). Thus, in the provision of domiciliary care services, old men and male carers may receive more services and receive them sooner, than old women or female carers.

Similar patterns also emerge in the admission of old men and old women to local authority residential care. Old men have tended to be admitted at an earlier age, and in better physical and mental health than women. Finally, although enforced loss of role activity involved in household management and self-care is more likely to affect the relatively large numbers of female residents who enter homes for older people, an understanding of the impact of this change is not reflected in the kinds of regime that prevail (Evans, Hughes and Wilkin 1981; Wilkin and Hughes 1987; Hughes and Wilkin 1987).

Implications for change: the development of radical practice

An attempt to develop a radical approach, based on principles of anti-discrimination, is a current theme in many areas of social work (Langan and Lee 1989). The processes of transforming good practice into radical practice, and of translating the principles of anti-discrimination into day-to-day work, are difficult enough for those areas of social work practice which have already achieved a degree of professional consensus around the definition of good enough practice. One of the major problems facing those who are attempting to develop anti-discriminatory practice with old people is the lack of a foundation of good practice principles upon which to build. Our objective here is to establish the principles upon which the development of anti-discriminatory practice could be based, and to then sketch out some implications for change.

First, social work practice must reflect an understanding of the oppressive impact of a capitalist, ageist and patriarchal society on all old women, but at the same time reject the stereotypical image of old women as passive victims. Second, social work practice must embody an understanding of the impact of ageism and sexism on all older women, but at the same time acknowledge the differentiation and heterogeneity derived from factors such as class, race and personal biography. Third, social work practice must challenge the discrimination which arises from ageism and sexism and yet continue to work in organizations whose policies towards old women reflect these values.

Thus, in helping individual old women to negotiate and improve the quality of their lives, anti-discriminatory social work practice has to struggle on a number of different fronts. These struggles are apparent at every stage of intervention and decision-making in the social work process, and at every level from the professional interaction with the individual older woman to the formulation of policy at the highest level.

Empowerment is a key concept in the translation of anti-discriminatory principles into policy and practice. At every point at which the social worker meets the conflict and contradictions inherent in the process of developing anti-discriminatory practice, the principle of empowerment of older women can help to negotiate a pathway through to new and qualitatively different practice. The concept of empowerment involves challenging the structured dependency of older women and must be derived from a knowledge and understanding of the principles we have discussed above. Phillipson (1989) has identified the need for campaigning work to challenge the material conditions of old age, for changes in the training of students as practitioners, and for the development of community-based initiatives to meet the needs of specific groups of older people, especially women and black people. However, while such developments are important, social workers also struggle to translate anti-discriminatory principles into their direct intervention in the lives of individual older women.

Direct social work encompasses a variety of tasks and skills, all of which could be significantly improved by the adoption of an anti-discriminatory perspective. For example, at the level of communication with older women, the way in which the practitioner approaches and talks to the older woman will reflect a belief in her right to respect and autonomy. There can be no place, then, for addressing old women by their first names without permission; for using infantilizing or stereotypical labels such as 'granny' or 'old dear'; for treating or speaking to the person in any way which symbolically reflects an abuse of power or an invasion of their privacy or rights. Development of anti-discriminatory practice at this very basic level also includes challenging ageist or sexist language used by colleagues, other members of staff, or other professionals.

The development of work with older people must begin by accepting that professional communication with older people is no less demanding than that with people from other client groups. Interaction with older women must involve all the general interviewing and communication skills intrinsic to good practice, as well as some specialist skills, knowledge and techniques relevant to older women. It is a reflection of the lack of status of work with older people, for example, that personal biography work is referred to as reminiscence, with connotations of misty romanticism and sentimentality, while with children it is called life story *work*.

Assessment processes need to encompass not only the needs and risks to which the older woman is subject, but also the strengths and resources derived from her whole-life experience. Assessment must be based on an understanding of the inferior structural position of older women, but it must articulate that understanding with the personal, economic, social, health, lifestyle and biographical characteristics of that particular older woman. The assessment must incorporate a detailed evaluation of the older woman herself – her health, social activities, functional abilities, critical life events, emotional state, relevant aspects of personal history, her financial and material conditions, her mood, her self-esteem. All of these factors must be examined to identify not only deficits or problems, but strengths and resources.

The assessment must also include the strengths and weaknesses of her familial and social relationships, her social network and contacts, her activity in and connections with her local community. Most importantly, the assessment must be conducted *with* the older woman. It must incorporate her views of her situation and her needs and yet not be limited by her low expectations and internalized acceptance of the consequences of ageism and sexism.

Some of the inherent tensions and contradictions of anti-discriminatory practice are brought into especially sharp relief during the assessment process. For example, a commitment to acknowledging and validating personal biography must not be a justification for intruding too deeply or too early into a woman's personal history. The commitment to assessing needs in a gender-sensitive as opposed to gender-biased way must not be a reason for ignoring the way old women themselves define their roles. The legitimate aim of raising the consciousness and expectations of old women must not be used to deny old women the right to determine their own futures and lifestyles.

Concluding remarks

In this chapter, we have tried to illuminate some of the political and professional issues which a radical social work practice with older people must confront. We have also begun to demonstrate how an analysis of practice at the level of direct work with older women leads to a detailed reappraisal and redefinition of how social workers execute their professional skills and tasks.

The development of a radical social work practice involves the challenging of discriminatory values and assumptions, many of which are deeply embedded in prevailing social, political and professional cultures. Phillipson (1989) has argued that this can only be achieved through social workers forging alliances with older people and their organizations. However, social workers also need to develop a support network within their own agencies, and the importance of team work, in generating the support and resources needed, must be recognized. This concept could refer not only to a team of social workers, but could also be a multi-discriplinary forum involving practitioners and users within a particular locality.

The development of a radical social work must begin with a critical analysis of current policy and practice at a local level, and a commitment to expose the discriminatory characteristics of existing service provision. For example, at the level of the team, the following questions could provide the framework for such an analysis:

- What are the age, sex and ethnic characteristics of the older people with whom we work?
- What kinds of services are most commonly offered to older people, compared to other client groups?
- Are different patterns of services discernible in relation to older women and older men?
- Are different patterns of services discernible in relation to female carers and male carers?

- How many older women from minority ethnic groups do we work with?
- Who in the team is working with older women and what is their level of skill/training?
- How is the team providing a voice for older women?
- What is our agency's policy on work with older people and how far does it acknowledge sources of discrimination?

The answers to some of these questions can provide a way forward to develop new policies and practices in relation to social work with older women at the level of the team. Dissemination of the answers and the proposed developments could begin a wider debate and process of change extending beyond the team.

Experience suggests that if those of us committed to developing anti-discriminatory social work with older people wait for initiatives to come from the highest policy-making levels within our agencies, many of us will wait a very long time. However, the development of radical policy and practice is a difficult and lonely task for the individual practitioner. The struggle, in our view, is one in which a corporate or collective approach is essential. Forming alliances with older people and their organizations is one element in this collective strategy. Another must be that social workers act together in their teams to examine their own values and practices, to challenge prevailing ageist policy and practice, and to take the initiative in instigating change.

References

Audit Commission (1985), *Managing Services for the Elderly More Effectively* (London: HMSO).

Bowl, R. (1986), 'Social work with old people', in C. Phillipson and A. Walker (eds), *Ageing and Social Policy: A Critical Assessment* (Aldershot: Gower) pp. 128–45.

Brody, E. M., Johnsen, P. T. and Fulcommer, M. C. (1984), 'What should adult children do for elderly parents: opinions and preferences of 3 generations of women', *Journal of Gerontology* 39, 6, pp. 736–46.

Bryan, B., Dadzie, S. and Scafe, S. (1985), *The Heart of the Race* (London: Virago Press).

Callender, C. (1987), 'Redundancy, unemployment and poverty', in C. Glendinning and J. Millar 1987, pp. 137–58.

Charlesworth, A., Wilkin, D. and Durie, A. (1984), *Carers and Services: A Comparison of Men and Women Caring for Dependent People* (Manchester: EOC).

Cumming, E. and Henry, W. E. (1961), *Growing Old* (New York: Basic Books).

Dominelli, L. (1989), *Anti-Racist Social Work* (London: Macmillan).

Evans, G., Hughes, B. and Wilkin, D. (1981), *The Management of Mental and Physical Impairment in Non-Specialist Residential Homes for the Elderly* Research Report 4 (Manchester: University of Manchester, Department of Psychiatry and Community Medicine).

Evers, H. (1983), 'Elderly women and disadvantage: perceptions of daily and support relationships', in D. Jerome (ed.), *Ageing in Modern Society* (London: Croom Helm) pp. 25–44.

Evers, H. (1985), 'The frail elderly woman: emergent questions in ageing and women's health', in E. Lewin and V. Olesen (eds), *Women, Health and Healing* (London: Tavistock) pp. 86–111.

Family Policy Studies Centre (1988), *An Ageing Population: Fact Sheet 2* (London: FPSC).

Fenton, S. (1988), 'Health, work and growing old: the Afro-Caribbean experience', *New Community* 15, 3, pp. 426–43.

Finch, J. (1984), 'Community care: developing non-sexist alternatives, *Critical Social Policy* 9, pp. 6–18.

Finch, J. and Groves, D. (1980), 'Community care and the family: a case for equal opportunities?' *Journal of Social Policy* 9, pp. 487–514.

Finch, J. and Groves, D. (eds) (1983), *A Labour of Love: Women, Work, and Caring* (London: Routledge and Kegan Paul).

Finch, J. and Groves, D. (1985), 'Old girl, old boy: gender divisions in social work with the elderly', in E. Brook and A. Davis (eds), *Women, the Family and Social Work* (London: Tavistock) pp 92–111.

Ford, G. and Taylor, R. (1981), 'Lifestyle and ageing', *Ageing and Society* 1, 3, pp. 329–45.

Ford, J. and Sinclair, R. (1987), *Sixty Years on: Women Talk about Old Age* (London: The Women's Press).

Ford, J. and Sinclair, R. (1989), 'Women's experience of old age', in P. Carter, T. Jeffs and M. Smith (eds), *Social Work and Social Welfare Yearbook 1* (Milton Keynes: Open University Press) pp. 74–90.

Gaffaney, P. (1988), 'Provision inadequate for ethnic communities', *Community Care* 10 March, p. 2.

Gamarnikow, E., Morgan, D. H. J., Purvis, J. and Taylorson, D. (1983), *The Public and the Private* (London: Heinemann).

Glendenning, F. (ed.) (1979), *The Elders in Ethnic Minorities* (Keele: The Beth Johnson Foundation, the Department of Adult Education University of Keele, and the Commission for Racial Equality).

Glendenning, F. and Pearson, M. (1988), *The Black and Ethnic Minority Elders in Britain: Health Needs and Access to Services* (Keele: Health Education Authority in Association with the Centre for Social Gerontology, University of Keele).

Glendinning, C. and Millar, J. (eds) (1987), *Women and Poverty in Britain* (Hemel Hempstead: Harvester Wheatsheaf).

Griffiths, R. (1988), *Community Care: Agenda for Action. A Report to the Secretary of State for Social Services* (London: HMSO).
Groves, D. (1987), 'Occupational pension provision and women's poverty in old age', in Glendinning and Millar 1987, pp. 199–220.

Hanmer, J. and Statham, D. (1988), *Women and Social Work* (London: Macmillan).
Hemmings, S. (1985), *A Wealth of Experience* (London: Pandora Press).
HMSO (1989), *Caring for People. Community Care in the Next Decade and Beyond.* Cmnd 849 (London: HMSO).
Hughes, B. and Wilkin, D. (1987), 'Physical care and quality of life in residential homes', *Ageing and Society* 7, pp. 399–425.
Hunt, A. (1978), *The Elderly at Home* (London: HMSO).

Langan, M. and Lee, P. (1989), *Radical Social Work Today* (London: Unwin Hyman).
Leonard, P. (1984), *Personality and Ideology: Towards a Materialist Understanding of the Individual* (London: Macmillan).

MacDonald, B. and Rich, C. (1984), *Look Me in the Eye* (London: The Women's Press).
Markides, K. S. (ed.) (1989), *Aging and Health* (Newbury Park: Sage).
Marshall, M. (1983), *Social Work with Old People* (London: Macmillan).
Matthews, S. H. (1979), *The Social World of Old Women* (Beverley Hills: Sage Publications).
Means, R. (1981), *Community Care and Meals on Wheels* Working Paper 21 (Bristol: University of Bristol, School for Advanced Urban Studies).
Mooneram, R. (1979), 'The Asian elders', in Glendenning 1979, pp. 50–3.

Norman, A. (1985), *Triple Jeopardy: Growing Old in a Second Homeland* (London: CPA).

OPCS (1982), *General Household Survey 1980* (London: HMSO).
OPCS (1983), *Census 1981: Persons of Pensionable Age* (London: HMSO).

Peace, S. (1986), 'The forgotten female: social policy and older women', in Phillipson and Walker 1986, pp. 61–86.
Phillipson, C. (1972), *Capitalism and the Construction of Old Age* (London: Macmillan).
Phillipson, C. (1989), 'Challenging dependency: towards a new social work with older people', in Langan and Lee 1989, pp. 192–207.
Phillipson, C. and Walker, A. (eds) (1986), *Ageing and Social Policy: A Critical Assessment* (Aldershot: Gower).

Rowlings, C. (1981), *Social Work with Elderly People* (London: George Allen and Unwin).

Stacey, M. (1983), 'Social sciences and the state: fighting like a woman', in Gamarnikow 1983, pp. 7–11.

Townsend, P. (1957), *The Family Life of Old People, An Inquiry in East London* (London: Routledge and Kegan Paul).
Townsend, P. (1979), *Poverty in the United Kingdom* (Harmondsworth: Penguin).
Townsend, P. (1981), 'The structured dependency of the elderly: a creation of social policy in the twentieth century', *Ageing and Society* 1, 1, pp. 5–28.
Townsend, P. and Davidson, N. (1988), *Inequalities in Health* (London: Pelican).
Tunstall, J. (1966), *Old and Alone: A Sociological Study of Old People* (London: Routledge and Kegan Paul).

Walker, A. (1981), 'Towards a political economy of old age', *Ageing and Society* 1, 1, pp. 73–94.
Walker, A. (1985), *The Care Gap: How can Local Authorities meet the Needs of the Elderly?* (London: Local Government Information Unit).
Walker, A. (1987), 'The poor relation: poverty among old women', in Glendinning and Millar 1987, pp. 178–98.
Whitehead, M. (1988), *The Health Divide* (London: Penguin).
Wilkin, D. and Hughes, B. (1987), 'Residential care of elderly people: the consumer's views', *Ageing and Society* 7, pp. 175–201.
Wright, F. D. (1986), *Left to Care Alone* (Aldershot: Gower).

Index